The Conduct of Care

The Conduct of Care

Understanding Nursing Practice

Joanna Latimer

**Blackwell
Science**

© 2000 by
Blackwell Science Ltd
Editorial Offices:
Osney Mead, Oxford OX2 0EL
25 John Street, London WC1N 2BL
23 Ainslie Place, Edinburgh EH3 6AJ
350 Main Street, Malden
    MA 02148 5018, USA
54 University Street, Carlton
    Victoria 3053, Australia
10, rue Casimir Delavigne
    75006 Paris, France

Other Editorial Offices:

Blackwell Wissenschafts-Verlag GmbH
Kurfürstendamm 57
10707 Berlin, Germany

Blackwell Science KK
MG Kodenmacho Building
7–10 Kodenmacho Nihombashi
Chuo-ku, Tokyo 104, Japan

The right of the Authors to be identified as
the Authors of this Work has been asserted
in accordance with the Copyright, Designs
and Patents Act 1988.

First published 2000

Set in 10/12.5 pt Sabon
by DP Photosetting, Aylesbury, Bucks
Printed and bound in Great Britain by
MPG Books Ltd, Bodmin, Cornwall

The Blackwell Science logo is a trade mark of
Blackwell Science Ltd, registered at the
United Kingdom Trade Marks Registry

DISTRIBUTORS

Marston Book Services Ltd
PO Box 269
Abingdon
Oxon OX14 4YN
(*Orders:* Tel: 01235 465500
          Fax: 01235 465555)

USA
Blackwell Science, Inc.
Commerce Place
350 Main Street
Malden, MA 02148 5018
(*Orders:* Tel: 800 759 6102
                781 388 8250
          Fax: 781 388 8255)

Canada
Login Brothers Book Company
324 Saulteaux Crescent
Winnipeg, Manitoba R3J 3T2
(*Orders:* Tel: 204 837 2987
          Fax: 204 837 3116)

Australia
Blackwell Science Pty Ltd
54 University Street
Carlton, Victoria 3053
(*Orders:* Tel: 03 9347 0300
          Fax: 03 9347 5001)

A catalogue record for this title is available
from the British Library

ISBN 0-632-05575-8

Library of Congress
Cataloging-in-Publication Data
Latimer, Joanna.
    The conduct of care : understanding
nursing practice/Joanna Latimer.
        p. ; cm.
    Includes bibliographical references and
index.
        ISBN 0-632-05575-8 (alk. paper)
    1. Geriatric nursing.   2. Nursing
assessment.   I. Title.
    [DNLM: 1. Geriatric Nursing.
2. Geriatric Assessment.   3. Nurse-
Patient Relations.   4. Nursing
Assessment.   WY 152 L3517c 2000]
RC954.L38 2000
610.73′65—dc21
                                00-036012

For further information on
Blackwell Science, visit our website:
www.blackwell-science.com

For my mother and my father

'... anything identified with practices that have a past runs the risk of being the "culture" that slows the impetus of innovation ... technology frees one from and economic competition must work free of the trammels of tradition. Culture is a drag.'

(Strathern, 1993, p. 19)

False happiness, since we know that we can use
Only the eye as faculty, that the mind
Is the eye, and that this landscape of the mind
Is a landscape only of the eye.

(Wallace Stevens, 1947)

'Curiosity is a vice that has been stigmatised in turn by Christianity, by philosophy, and even by a certain conception of science. Curiosity is seen as futility. However, I like the word; it suggests something quite different to me. It "evokes" care; it is the care one takes of what exists and what might exist...'

(Foucault, 1980, p. 328)

Contents

Preface

The *Conduct of Care* draws on an ethnography of the bedside of older people admitted as emergencies to an acute medical unit. Nurses' assessment and care of these elderly people formed the focus of the study. Extensive discussion of nursing assessment, the care of acutely ill older people and the study's methodology can be found in Appendices 1, 2 and 3, respectively.

The book rediscovers the relationship between nurses' conduct, the politics of contemporary health care and a professionalising agenda. In summary, it explores the contemporary themes of:

- The scope and purpose of nursing practice
- The constitution of nurses' knowledge
- The constituents of quality in an acute care context

Chapter 2 describes the hospital, patients and staff to show how the multiple agendas which nurses face are made present in their day-to-day lives. Nurses are faced by organisational arrangements which have the potential to industrialise the hospital, to turn patients into an object that is to be processed. These arrangements focus nurses on a patient's discharge, reinforcing specialisation and potentially narrowing the scope of nursing concerns. For nurses, these agendas are potentially incompatible with the call from the profession for the nurture and care of the individual in all his needs. Nurses square their accounts by aligning themselves with the third agenda made present in everything they do: the demands coming from the need to maintain the space where first class medicine is available.

Chapter 3 examines how nursing processes organise and order ward life. Nursing handovers, ward routines, nursing records and the use of space and time act in concert to manage ward life and help accomplish the multiple demands coming from managerial, medical and professional agendas. So, while it is clear that the organisation of a ward depends upon nurses, nurses are not free to do whatever they will. Nurses are the conductors of care, but their conduct is restrained.

Chapter 4 examines consultant ward rounds and the social round.

Nurses' work of contextualising patients' troubles and monitoring their progress provides some of the grounds for moving patients through the medical domain. Medicine emerges as a resource which requires distribution, and as a practice in which both nurses and doctors engage. But the chapter also shows how the bedside is a space of performance through which a particular kind of medicine is produced and reproduced. Because of the way ward rounds are conducted, nurses' organising work is effaced at the same time as it contributes to the flow of beds. The ward round emerges then as the spectacle through which first class medicine is recreated as central to the work of the medical domain. At the same time, nurses' 'dirty work' of organising ward life is put back-stage.

Chapter 5 describes how nurses conduct their encounters with patients. It focuses on how nurses organise the period of time when a patient arrives on the ward, and immediately after. Nurses' conduct of the admission period initiates patients into the social organisation of the medical domain. Through their encounters with nurses, patients learn how to conduct themselves to maintain their inclusion as clinical materials. Critically, patients (like nurses) must efface themselves as social beings to be rendered appropriate to the medical domain. This includes allowing others to authorise their needs. Patients learn that 'authority', to define what is significant and to legitimate action, lies far from the bedside, not in the nurse–patient relationship. So that the bedside emerges not as the centre of discretion; discretion lies in other bodies of knowledge. But through the nurse–patient relationship some patients maintain their inclusion as appropriate medical materials.

Chapter 6 examines nurses' accounts. This brings into the debate not just how they think and work, but what it is that makes up a good and valuable hospital from a nurse's perspective. While nurses, like doctors, draw on medical discourse as the key method for making sense of patients' troubles and of legitimating their own activities, they have extended the medical gaze. Nurses go far beyond drawing on biomedical understandings to make their assessments of patients' needs. They describe themselves as proficient at reading a patient's social history and observing their behaviour to contextualise their troubles as well as monitor their progress. Through nursing accounts the constituting of classes is affirmed, and nurses technologise their understandings of patients to institute a nursing gaze. These accounts refigure the bedside as the space of observation through which nurses extend their lines of sight to include all aspects of patients – clinical, personal as well as psychosocial.

Chapter 7 completes the book with a summary and discussion of the implications for notions of care, for patients, for research on nursing efficacy and for the education, recruitment and retention of nurses.

In summary, *The Conduct of Care* is intended as an evocation of ward life. The objective is to resonate with nurses' own experiences of the dilemmas and complexity of practising in today's health service. In doing this, I hope the book takes its readers on a journey, one which transforms their understanding of the hospital – the space in a nurse's conduct of care. The path followed is a new one, one intended to make the experience of the original landscape irrecoverable. Any journey which takes the reader through a detailed presentation and analysis of the ethnographic material is integral to its arrival.

I have debated at length whether to include the extensive methodological and philosophical discussion from my thesis as a separate account in the book. I thought that treating this theoretical framework, which draws on a mixture of different contemporary social theories, separately from the analysis would impede the reading of the ethnography. It is in this regard that, with the exception of Appendix 3 and some of the footnotes, the methodological and theoretical underpinnings of the analysis are implicit to the ideas that the book offers. Where appropriate, I have referenced publications which contain more explicit theoretical discussion for any reader who would like to pursue this aspect.

Finally, I would like to acknowledge certain influences and sources of support that helped me while I prepared this book. In Lyotard's words I am a post, through which messages pass and translations are made. First, I was given a Scottish Home and Health Department Nursing Research Training Fellowship for two years which launched me on my present career. The work I did during that time formed the basis of this study. Second, the study was one of several undertaken at Edinburgh at the same time. I am not sure why so many interesting studies of nursing took place at that time, but they did, and while we have all gone our separate ways, we are in touch and I hope that our work is beginning to make a contribution, not just within nursing, but also to other disciplines, and to more general understanding about research, health, illness and the health professions.

While there were many people who have had an affect on the book I would specifically like to thank the following. Alison Tierney for her patience, common sense and tolerance, and Tom McGlew for his support in the early days. John Holmwood for opening me up to the world of social theory and argument, and Tony Cohen for his faith in the work and in me. Other students who informed and helped my thinking include Carl May, Maxine Mueller and Mary Ellen Purkis, whose own studies are all marvellous pieces of work.

I cannot thank enough all the patients, their families, doctors, nurses and other staff with whom I have worked, as well as those who are the actors in my ethnography, for giving me their time and for letting me into their worlds so trustingly. Thanks also to my publisher, Griselda Campbell, whose encouragement gave me the final push I needed to rewrite the book.

As academics we all need intellectual recognition and succour. I express my appreciation to all those people who have both encouraged me as well as contributed to my understanding. These include Nick Lee, Judith Parker, Anne Marie Rafferty, Trudy Rudge and Jan Savage – all of you have helped me in ways which are invaluable. Jane Robinson, who examined the thesis upon which this book is based, and David Silverman, who reviewed my first sociological paper, continue as valued colleagues and advocates. I would also like to acknowledge Marilyn Strathern, for her support, but also because her own work plays profound parts in my analysis in ways which cannot always be made explicit. Finally, my love and appreciation go to my husband, Rolland Munro, who is not only my greatest champion but whose work is a continual source of illumination, and to my two children, Jamie and Arabella.

The study has been theorised in the following publications by the author.

The nursing process re-examined: diffusion or translation? *Journal of Advanced Nursing* 22 213–20 (1995)

Giving patients a future: the constituting of classes in an acute medical unit. *Sociology of Health and Illness* 19(2) 160–85 (1997)

Older people in hospital: the labour of division. Affirmation and the stop (1997). In *Ideas of Difference: Social Spaces and the Labour of Division* (K. Hetherington & R. Munro, eds), pp. 273–97. Sociological Review Monograph. Blackwell, Oxford.

Figuring identities: older people, medicine and time (1997). In *Critical Approaches to Ageing and Later Life* (A. Jamieson, S. Harper & C. Victor), pp. 143–59. Open University Press, Milton Keynes.

Organising context: nurses' assessments of older people in an acute medical unit. *Nursing Inquiry* 5(1) 43–57 (1998)

The dark at the bottom of the stair: participation and performance of older people in hospital. *Medical Anthropology Quarterly* 13(2) 186–213 (1999)

Robinson, J., Avis, M., Latimer, J. & Traynor, M. (1999). *Interdisciplinary Perspectives on Health Policy and Practice. Competing Interests or Complementary Interpretations?* Churchill Livingstone, Edinburgh.

Socialising disease: medical categories and inclusion of the aged. *Sociological Review* 48 (in press).

Becoming a Reflective Practitioner
Christopher Johns
0-632-05561-8

Based on everyday clinical practice, this text shows that reflective practice is a dynamic process which evolves as the practitioner develops his or her own practice. The examples used guide the reader through the stages of reflective practice in the context of the caring relationship with the client.

Transforming Nursing through Reflective Practice
Edited by Christopher Johns and Dawn Freshwater
0-632-04784-4

This book looks at the transformation of nursing through practice, education, and research connected with this fast growing interest within nursing. Ideas within this book will be a rich source of information and guidance to help practitioners explore a range of well tried approaches to achieving meaningful reflective practice.

Successful Supervision in Health Care Practice: Promoting Professional Development
Edited by Jenny Spouse and Liz Redfern
0-632-05159-0

This text provides answers about how to implement supervision successfully and how to survive as a supervisor. There is a strong theoretical and research base throughout the book that offers an approach to learning in practice.

Mentoring, Preceptorship and Clinical Supervision: A Guide to Professional Support Roles in Clinical Practice
Second Edition
Alison Morton-Cooper and Anne Palmer
0-632-04967-7

Introducing learning support systems into clinical practice is a major issue for today's health professional. This book will stimulate fresh thinking about what we need and can gain from professional learning support. It challenges professionals to recognise the value of support in promoting trust and collegiality within the diverse settings used to promote learning health care.

Reflective Practice in Nursing: The Growth of the Professional Practitioner
Second Edition
Edited by Sarah Burns and Chris Bulman
0-632-05291-0

This second edition has responded to the increasing interest amongst nurses to master the skills of reflective practice. It offers a motivating and accessible text that documents and analyses the increase in knowledge and skills surrounding the subject.

Chapter 1

Setting the Scene: The Complexity of Nursing Practice

Background to the study

'Medical nursing is (also) highly skilled work... The physician's diagnosis must rest upon the careful observation of symptoms over time
where the surgeon's are in larger part dependent on visible things. *The
lack of visibility creates problems on the medical.* A patient will see his
nurse stop at the next bed and chat for a moment or two with the patient
there. He doesn't know that she is observing the shallowness of the
breathing and colour and tone of skin. He thinks she is just visiting. So,
alas, does his family who may thereupon decide that these nurses aren't
very impressive. If the nurse spends more time at the next bed than his
own, the patient may feel slighted... The nurses are "wasting time"
unless they are darting about doing some visible thing such as administering hypodermics.' (Lentz, 1954, cited in Goffman, 1958, p. 20)

Imagine the scale of the problem here. Nurses' work is rational, skilled
and evidence-based. But it doesn't appear like that. What patients and
their relatives see is nurses chatting. At the very moment when nurses may
be carrying out a diagnosis or medical check, they appear to be doing
something else – 'wasting time'.

What should nurses do about this? Should they abandon their uniforms
for the white coats of doctors, and adopt the grave faces of lawyers and
accountants? The *Conduct of Care* explores these tensions. I stationed
myself at the bedside to record nurses' talk and observe the 'invisible'
work that accompanies it. I joined nurses on their handovers and shared
coffee on their breaks, and I talked to nurses and patients to find out how
each saw the world they were helping to create. This ethnography is as
much their story as it is mine.

But this is not all the book is about. I also followed nurses as they
responded to demands to reduce waiting times and make their work
'efficient'. In short, I have been following nurses as they attempt to make

their work more 'visible'. So this is also the story of a National Health Service under strain.

The book evokes the complexity of nursing practice in today's health services. It makes clear how medicine is distributed between nurses and doctors, but it also makes visible what is usually effaced, even by nurses themselves: that it is nurses' conduct of care which produces ward life.

The book proposes that without nurses' complex organisation of ward life there would be no hospitals, and no NHS. But nurses are not free to conduct care however they will; present in nurses' everyday lives are the potentially competing agendas of medicine, professionalisation and health policy.

The Conduct of Care draws on an ethnography of the bedside of older people admitted as emergencies to an acute medical unit in a prestigious UK teaching hospital. The impetus for the study stemmed from several concerns. First, I was concerned over the precarious position of older people in health care environments. While older people are more likely to become ill and have complex effects from their illness than people from other age groups, paradoxically, they are not necessarily welcome in the acute medical domain. This paradox was exemplified for me as a medical Ward Sister, when a medical registrar, telephoning me to say that he had a new admission, apologised because she was 'an 85-year-old woman with a massive stroke'. When I said to send her up because that was 'what we were there for', he responded with 'Oh, I forgot, you're the Sister who likes old people'.

The assessment and care of older people in the acute sectors of health services, in any part of the world, is a critical site for research because it brings to the surface problems and difficulties about culture and representation, not just of older people, but also of what is valued and worthy in a Euro-American context. For example, the care of ill older people is increasingly considered a burden on health care services because it is characterised as a drain on precious resources. The burden is rapidly being shifted onto other, non-professional shoulders, and this mobility relies on the institution of a division between health-related troubles which require the services of health professionals, and those which require the services of others. Nurses are trained and educated to believe that they should attend to all a person's needs deriving from their health troubles. Narrowing the purpose and meaning of hospital care down to the diagnosis and treatment of acute illness has important implications for nursing. The question arises: how are nurses dealing with this potential conflict? And how do they feel about it?

A second set of concerns revolves around what is happening to the practices of nurses and doctors more generally, and the relationship between them. Under change agendas which stress value for money and efficiency, health professionals are positioned to compete with each other and to justify their practices. But what counts for purposeful work is increasingly prescribed by agendas which lie outside traditional professional values. In its quest for professional status, I see nursing as embracing individualism and following the doctors in the abandonment of the bedside. This situation is not the nurses' fault; on the contrary, I hope that this book helps to show how nurses themselves are caught in intricate webs where the performance of professional identity has its own politics and logic.

The third set of concerns emerged as the study progressed. These concerns related to ideas of knowledge. There was the problem of 'bumping up against facts', and the even stranger problem of their disappearance at the very moment when one expects to bump against them. In particular, it seemed to me that there were certain things that were more likely to be taken notice of in acute care contexts than others, such as facts, whereas things like feelings, for example, were more likely to be ignored. During my research for this book I gradually developed a way to understand that all facts are indeed produced through processes of representation, and that these processes both construct the fact and mediate its interpretation. This is not to devalue facts. Rather, it helps to suggest that all evidence is on tenuous ground, and that a critical part of our work can be to try to both cross-check our facts and also to attempt to understand why some 'evidence' seems to resist refutation, and stands more firmly than others.

A fourth set of concerns are connected to a strange phenomenon within nursing itself: how within nursing theory there is a pervasive assumption that there are always better ways to do nursing. It seems to me that nursing theorists and many researchers continually go to other theories (such as cognitive psychology) and try to make nursing fit them, instead of going to nursing practice and make nursing not like other things but like itself, and *then* try to understand it. One of the problems with this is, of course, that there is not 'a thing' called nursing. Nursing is precisely local and specific, not standardised, and nursing can be many things: hesitant, incomplete, decisive, objective, subjective, concerned with dirt, with science and technology, with the heroic and the mundane, with bodies and with emotion and with thinking. Nursing is indeed that worst of all creatures in modernity, a hybrid. And even worse than this, it is a hybrid which occupies a peculiar space, the in-between. Nursing has to continually change and metamorphose to fit into spaces which are often shaped by forces other than its own – the space made by a disease in someone's life; the space left by a doctor as he leaves a patient puzzled by his explanation; the space left by a heart which has stopped and needs to be restarted again.

Theorists and researchers who strive to standardise nursing by continually reaching for standards or norms from elsewhere seem to me to miss the point. For example, many researchers and commentators on health service operations think that the magic bullet for improving patient care is better communication. Underlying this view there is an assumption that nurses are either bad communicators or do not communicate.

'There seems little doubt that nurses do not generally communicate with their patients.' (Faulkner, 1985)

In this book, a much less dogmatic view is taken of what might constitute good or bad communication. By taking a less normative view, it emerges that doctors, nurses, patients, and other things in the world are, indeed, communicating *all the time*. But the question arises over how nurses are communicating, what their methods and strategies for communicating accomplish, and, probably most importantly, why might they be accomplishing those particular things rather than other things at any one moment. Making nursing visible depends on developing methods unfamiliar to nursing theory or health services research. In this respect, my own approach is to understand the communicative practices of nurses, patients and doctors at the bedside as an effect of (and as affecting) wider sociocultural relations as well as shifts in health policy.

Ahead of the chapters, I should add that the research resists the temptation to either heroise or damn. Some of what I saw amounts to 'bad practice for good organisational reasons' (Garfinkel, 1967), while other aspects of nurses conduct seemed angelic, even saintly. But I see no good coming from glorifying what nurses do as angelic. I saw my task rather as that of helping nurses to gain a better understanding of how their *own* conduct contributes to the organisation and delivery of health care. A better understanding of the complexities of what it is that nurses do can help them press for more trust in their abilities. The over-riding aim of the book is therefore to help nurses articulate their distinctions so that they can care for patients in ways that limit hospitals from becoming inhuman spaces of indifference.

The invisibility of nursing

Visibility is first of all about visual perception. For example, Lentz points to the easy visibility of surgical nurses:

'The things which a nurse does for post-operative patients on the surgical floor are frequently of recognisable importance, even to patients who are strangers to hospital activities. For example, the patient sees his nurse changing bandages, swinging orthopaedic frames into place, and can realise that these are purposeful activities.' (Lentz, 1954)

Trust and visibility, it seems, go hand in hand. Yet what people are actually doing is never transparent in itself. Care is made 'visible' through the use of *signs*, the bandages and the orthopaedic frames.

According to the influential writings of the sociologist Erving Goffman (1958, p. 21), people use signs to 'dramatise' aspects of what they do. The above extracts, which Goffman quotes from Lentz, illustrate how nurses might have difficulties dramatising other aspects of their work. Medical nurses, in particular, appear to lack the sign equipment with which to make their purposes explicit. Care is not all dispensing drugs and giving bed baths and much of what they do remains invisible.

Visibility stands, then, for a 'way of seeing'. So this means that visibility is a term which is also metaphorical. It refers to an understanding which is *interpretative*: visibility happens when the work that people do appears to others as rational, sensible and appropriate. Problems arise today, for both nurses and patients, because the work nurses do is no longer being taken for granted. The demand on all hospital workers is for everyone to justify – make visible – what they do. But if nurses lack the sign equipment which a patient can read, their conduct easily becomes *in*visible. And when patients no longer understand what the nurse is doing, conditions are ripe for them to feel they are experiencing a lack of care: *the nurses should do more!*

The bedside

Traditionally, the bedside of the sick is treated as a simple location. It is the site of nurture, comfort and care. The bed is a place of rest and restitution, suffering and death. Nurses are the alleviators of pain and suffering, supportive and comforting to the sick. Indeed, the etymology of nurse is 'nurturer'.

But nurses are not just nurturers: their conduct today must meet with the demands of a professionalising agenda. Most models of nursing, even if they stress different objectives, press the traditional view towards that of negotiation and decision making. Many nursing models give the impression that it is up to nurses to decide how they conduct care at the bedside. Specifically, they represent nurses as engaged in one-to-one relations, privileging individual patients' needs and seeing them as whole people. More recently, nursing theorists have emphasised that patients' views and meanings should inform care so that decisions about needs and care are to be mutually negotiated and agreed with the patient.

These different motifs of nurture and negotiation resonate with the everyday experiences of nurses in contemporary health service contexts (for example, Davies, 1995). Stressing the bedside as a space of democratised relations acknowledges the extent to which meanings of care have become contestable and this renders the bedside more complicated. Within these new views of care, the implied failure of nurses to treat patients as competent agents or sentient individuals has been attributed to the context of health care, lack of skill or knowledge, the emotionally difficult nature of nursing work, or to medical dominance. There is something in all of this. But, as explanations of practice, they do not help nurses explain what it is exactly that their practices *do* in fact accomplish.

The first aim of this book is to illustrate how explanations offered by nursing models underplay the complexity of the bedside. For example, nurses and patients are not free to negotiate the space at the bedside however they want. Indeed, constraints on conduct are many and intense. Conduct is prescribed by ethical codes and hospital rules, it is sedimented by traditions and procedures and constrained by the demands of many other activities. Yet, as the examples in the book show, nurses accomplish their multiple agendas, both by drawing on codes, rules, traditions and procedures and by surpassing them.

The scope of nursing practice

Nurses' conduct must continuously pass the test of visibility. As we have seen, there is a relationship between the scope of nurses' practices, the pressure for nurses to make their work visibly purposeful and the easy visibility of nursing work which is either technical or in support of medical interventions.

What passes for work at the bedside is always being constituted through a complex range of associations. The associations reflect wider socio-cultural matters, such as the demand for improvement in medical research and efficiency in service. For example, Lentz (1954) treated the bedside as a *social space*, but also as a space of surveillance. Although the bedside is a place from which patients make sense of nurses' conduct, it is the place within which their bodies are administered and observed. Therefore the bedside is a space through which patients themselves are being made visible to the medical gaze, otherwise why are they there, taking up valuable resources?

Nurses are also under surveillance, not least by themselves. For example, purposeful work for nurses requires outcomes which are clear and distinct. This demand for clear and distinct outcomes derives not only more recently from managerial agendas, but also from their association with medical work. It is medical work which makes nurses' practices distinct from what other women do, regularly and without pay. What this means is that conduct which is efficacious and clinical is seen to entail sticking to the medical aspects of the nurses' work and playing down what seem to be 'social' practices like talking to patients.

The bedside is best considered as a socially constructed location in which some things are being made present, while others are made absent. For example, while the hospital bedside is valorised as a place for the acutely ill, the social is denigrated by everyone concerned. In Lentz's example, what won't do is chatting. Instead, for both nurses and patients alike, what gives visibility to nurses is their use of medical discourse.

Contested interests

Lentz's study was published in 1954 and Goffman's in 1958. What is interpreted today to be rational, skilled or evidence-based conduct at the bedside is influenced by much more than the patient's or a theoretical view of nursing. There are two further views which also have an effect. First, there is the irritation of the manager as to whether the nurses' visits to the bed are in any way related to his goals – measurable outcomes and increased throughput. Second, there is the doctor whose own clinical performance rests upon having the right kinds of patients in the beds.

Contemporary health policy, concerned with service outcomes and increased accountability for cost as well as care, has refigured the bed as a commodity and the bedside as a space of *production*. This means that permissible conduct at the bedside is affected by the demands of the new management, which applies new sets of tools for making work at the bedside visible. These new management tools are those provided by accountants and auditors. Under their pressures, the question of who (or what) gets to decide who has access to the bed (and all that goes with it) is no longer the prerogative of nurses and doctors; it is continually negotiated and contested (see also Green & Armstrong, 1993). Further, it is not just the presence of patients that has to be justified; all the work around them has also to be made visible. Specifically, nurses' work has to be visible to managers to justify expenditure. It has to be rational, skilled and evidence-based from the managers' perspective, not just from that of the profession. Nurses now have to show managers that their work is more than women's work *and* different from the work of doctors.

Turning to the demands of the medical profession, the bedside is not just the space from which the patient is administered and observed, as in Lentz's study. The bedside is also a space of performance. Medicine as a research-based discipline is performed through a distribution of practices between nurses and doctors, and between the bedside and the ward round.

But in order for medicine to accomplish its own objectives and dramatise its own visibility as applied research, it requires particular kinds of patients, and not all patients will do.

The bedside, then, is not simply the site of care. It is the site of organisational politics. The bedside today is made complex by the interests of managers and doctors. Within this context, measuring nurses' conduct against the profession's calls to impose their discretion at the bedside seems almost inane. In contrast, treating the bedside as a complex location allows new understandings about nurses' accomplishments to come into view – nurses organise the bedside in line with much more than the demands of the professional discourses of nurturing and negotiation.

Nurses organising the bedside

This book addresses what is almost completely absent from contemporary theories. It draws attention to how nurses's conduct orders and organise ward life. As well as revealing the enormous range of skills that make up the complexity of nursing practice, the analysis details how nurses' conduct does much more than deliver care to individual patients.

In the following chapters, the bedside is treated as a complex, sedimented location. Nurses are not, despite many professional and theoretical accounts which stress their individual accountability, free to do whatever they will. Nurses are seen here as the conduits through which the complex and conflicting demands of current health and professional policy are accomplished and translated at the bedside.

The aim of the book is to remind nurses of all the work they do – both that which is downgraded and effaced and that which is highlighted and encouraged. My objective is to begin to reground the theoretical and policy debate about nursing. In order to align the conduct of nurses with managerial demands for clarity and distinction, nurse educationalists and policy makers have reached for technologies: sometimes complex ones like the 'nursing process', sometimes more simplistic ones like the 'named nurse'. The effects of these moves have been to consolidate the bedside as a site of surveillance.

In summary, contemporary nurses practise in a context influenced by several key debates:

• Nursing as a profession
• Accountability for nurses
• The efficiency and effectiveness of nursing practice
• Quality of care
• What counts as rational, skilled and evidence-based practice.

These debates have mainly been driven by the agendas of nurse educationalists, the professional nursing bodies, health policy advisors and health service managers. They put pressure on nurses to:

- Fall into line with traditional models of professional expertise, which narrow the forms of evidence upon which practice can be justified
- Agree to the individuation of their accountability
- Engage in the demands of managers for proof of a demonstrable gain from nursing care
- Improve service efficiency.

In contrast, *The Conduct of Care* addresses these debates from the perspectives of practising nurses.

Chapter 2

Organisation of Care within the Hospital Setting

Introduction

Nurses accomplish many things. Some effects are quite unexpected and will be discussed later. Specifically this chapter focuses on the main ways in which nurses can be considered to *organise* the hospital. In terms of organisation, nurses have three day-to-day concerns:

- Preserving the quality of acute medicine
- Managing the flow of patients through the beds
- Getting care to patients.

Critically, the chapter takes the view that organisation is not the result of people alone. Key organisational artefacts, such as the ward round and the waiting system, help to keep these three concerns present in the everyday lives of nurses.

Royal University Hospital: first class medicine in a third world environment

Royal University Hospital is a monument to a particular tradition: British medicine. The hospital is located in the heart of an historic city. It was purpose built in the late nineteenth century, next to the even older, renowned medical school.

The hospital's main entrance consists of elegant mahogany doors, a floor of marble tiles, and walls bedecked with large, dark portraits, and wooden panels engraved with names in gold, representing the eminent physicians and surgeons who have practised there. Almost no-one uses this entrance. There are many ways in and out of the hospital, so tradition is easily passed by. Most people come into the hospital through its side entrances. These consist of flapping pairs of plastic doors which admit patients, staff and families into long, high and draughty corridors with linoleum floors and bare walls. A sense of desolation and dirt is evoked by the cigarette butts on the ground outside.

The hospital has a dual identity. The front entrance announces that this is the clinical setting for the internationally prestigious and historic medical faculty. The side entrances remind one that this is a regional, National Health Service (NHS) hospital, where medical care is free to almost all comers. So, while the hospital is archaic and inconvenient in its lofty Victorian architecture, and perpetually short of money and space, it is none the less figured, as the Professor of Medicine put it to me, as where 'first class medicine' is practised albeit 'in a third world environment'.

The hospital is not, then, just a place for the sick to get well, but also for large numbers of students to get educated and qualified. It is also where those already qualified maintain and further their expertise, experience and, critically, their professional identities.

Medicine as spectacle

While their clients include people from every social group, the rich and the poor alike, many of the practitioners who work in the hospital are committed to maintaining a performance of formality, eminence and, importantly, altruism. Hospital practitioners, then, are not just engaged in being identified as members of their various professions. Instead, Royal University Hospital is also a 'spectacle' – a space in which practitioners are continuously performing and reproducing British medicine as a prestigious, eminent and non-commercial institution.

Consultants' ward rounds, therefore, are formal and spectacular occasions for exercising and passing on medicine. People from all over the world may attend these occasions so that sometimes there are up to twenty people, all in white, gathered around a bed or a notes trolley to watch and participate in the performance and recreation of medicine.

But, as will emerge, this is an NHS under strain. So too is the practice of first class medicine which depends upon the presence of appropriate patients. Thus, an aspect of the performance of first class medicine is the concern to maintain the *purity* of medicine (Latour, 1991), and this purity is under threat.

Throughout the rest of this book the restricted space in which first class medicine is performed will be referred to as 'the clinical domain'. Like the original entrance hall, the clinical domain of first class medicine has become surrounded by leaky spaces so that the purity of the clinical domain entails continuous labour by practitioners, and surprisingly, by many patients.

The wards

Royal University Hospital is divided into different sectors, each with its own structures and administrative support. These include a surgical and medical directorate and, within these, there are different units consisting usually of four single-sex wards each. These in turn are broken down into pairs of parallel wards, each pair having a responsibility for general medicine and for providing some specialisms.

A 'ward' consists of a bounded space and has its own amenities, such as a kitchen, lavatories and bathrooms, treatment room, drug, equipment and linen stores, patients' sitting room, secretaries', doctors' and nurses' offices, and various divisions in which beds and lockers are located. These latter divisions consist of a main ward area, side rooms and cubicles. The main ward areas are open plan and are partitioned into four bays (1 to 4), with each bay consisting of four or five beds. The 'nurses' station' is in the middle of the ward. The ward structure can be considered a crude panopticon (Foucault, 1976), through which patients and nurses alike are under surveillance and exposed to gaze.

This form of facility is common in British hospitals, and can be seen as helping to mark how the observation of illness and its treatment takes precedence over notions of privacy, as well as how there are constant constraints imposed by limited resources. The provision of single rooms, for example, is usually untenable given NHS budgets.

Signs and charts

The medical unit in which the fieldwork for this study took place is the professorial medical unit. It consists of a female and a male ward, each containing between 28 and 30 beds. Each bed space has a bed, a locker and curtains, which are hung so that each bed can be screened off. On the head of each bed is a holder for a name card. These cards are colour coded for each consultant and have the patient's names written on them (their title and surname, sometimes their forename as well, or just their forename and surname and no title). The patients are not a party to the colour coding of their name cards, they are not given the key to the code to know that pink means 'under the care of Dr X'. So while the cards help staff identify patients within the setting, the card does not allow patients mutual identification of their place within the setting, i.e. to know under whose care they are.

Also hanging on the wall above the bed is an observation chart. The patient's name is written on this as well as recordings of temperature, pulse, blood pressure, respiration and occasionally bowel movements. The public display of this personal information is taken for granted by staff as facilitating easy identification of patients and access to basic information. For example, porters and physiotherapists do not have to approach nursing staff to locate patients nor do they have to be introduced to patients. They walk around the wards looking at the name cards until they find the person they are looking for.

At one level these arrangements mean patients are open to a wider variety of 'personnel' to whom they do not need to be 'formally' introduced by a member of ward staff who is already known. Rather, they can be approached directly. But this also means that patients are more exposed. Anyone can approach them so there is no protection such as that which more formal arrangements provide. Another feature of these arrangements is that they lead to less contact between personnel and a reduction in opportunities for casual encounter and discussion. This in turn may minimise the flow of information between department and ward personnel over a patient's response or progress.

The charts also mean that nurses and doctors do not have to memorise names and faces as assiduously as in a situation where identifying information is not on display. Under these circumstances, the face as an identifying feature may not come to matter so much; patients can be identified by the signs constructed to represent them and the face does not have to be attended to in the same way for recognition to occur. Where nurses work very closely with someone on a regular basis, this will not necessarily be the case. They know the patient by their face and can recognise them wherever they are in the ward. But as longer lengths of stay become a feature of the past, nurses need to have ways of easily remembering who patients are.

These details of ward organisation help to constitute the social relationships between patients and staff: patients are more exposed and less well defended by old conventions, but they are also more accessible. Further, by breaching traditional ideas about confidentiality and dignity, such organisational arrangements emphasise the more functional and streamlined aspects of the service – patients are not here to stay, they are here to be observed and worked on, and cured or relieved of the effects of disease.

While these procedures may appear to subordinate privacy, dignity and confidentiality to expediency and convenience, they also symbolise another aspect of ward life. The public display of personal information is one of the ways in which patients are inducted into the orders of the setting. The charts and the writing upon them represent aspects of the patient made visible through the medical gaze. Features of patients inscribed in hieroglyphics on charts become the nurses' and doctors' materials for the production of a purely clinical domain. Charts allow nurses to make their activities visible and seen as purposeful and disciplined. This theme, of transforming the patient into a medical object, is returned to throughout the book.

Ward personnel

The wards each have their own complement of nursing staff, headed by a ward sister. During the study the nursing staff complement for each ward varied over time but included six permanent qualified nurses (one sister* and five staff nurses), between seven and twelve students at various stages of their training, and two nursing auxiliaries. Each of the staff nurses rotated onto night duty opposite a night staff nurse who worked alternative weeks. Of the forty or so nurses in the study, all but one staff nurse, one student nurse and a nursing auxiliary were women.

The two wards shared a senior nurse who held unit meetings (she was responsible for four wards altogether), so the wards were administered as a unit by nursing administration. The senior nurse visited the wards twice a day and checked the numbers of staff. An important aspect of her visits was to ascertain the potential numbers of empty beds. She usually stayed by the nurses' station during her visit and sometimes chatted with the nurse-in-charge. Typically the senior nurse did not have anything to do with the patients directly nor did she audit how they were being nursed. Ward nurses were expected to self-regulate their work in line with hospital policies and procedures. They were judged by nursing administration on their ability to control the environment, the absence of complaints (from patients, doctors and the nursing school), and their capacity to deliver free beds at the right time. The senior nurses were therefore no longer intermediaries, placing themselves somewhere between the needs of the service and the needs of individual patients. They are now firmly placed in the management line, not the clinical.

The wards also shared the same doctors. Each of the four consultant physicians attached to the unit had a team of doctors working under him. At the time of the study, all the doctors except one female resident were men. The doctors above resident level had responsibilities which took them to other departments. Almost all of the middle grade and more senior physicians were employed by both the university and the health service so that many of them were university lecturers and researchers as well as clinicians. The patients were both their research and their teaching material.

---

* In British nursing 'sister' indicates a female charge nurse. Student nurses were still not supernumerary at the time of study.

Other people working in the wards included a housekeeper, domestic cleaners, occupational therapists, physiotherapists, a medical social worker, dieticians, a speech therapist, and a chaplain. There were facilities outside the ward to which patients could be taken: a physiotherapy department, an occupational therapy department and a chapel, but much of the work of these departments actually took place in the wards themselves. In this way members of these other departments were present in the wards, some more than others. Social work, for example, was a relatively scarce resource and the presence of the social worker was equally scarce. In contrast, physiotherapists and occupational therapists were present on the wards more often.

Identity and accountability

All qualified medical and nursing staff at the Royal University Hospital wear white. This traditional practice exemplifies how clinical identity is portrayed, not just as purity and cleanliness, but also as an effacement of the wearer: individuality, self-interest and the social are effaced through the plainness of uniformity.

The two wards did not 'act together' as a unit. The Sisters did not have regular meetings together, the wards did not share staff nor did the ward nurses have the opportunity to share ideas, feelings, or discuss their work. Patients did not mix, and only minimal amounts of equipment were shared between the wards, such as heparin pumps. Informally, the nurses did not 'have much to do with one another' (Sister, field notes, Ward 2) and occasions like 'ward nights out' were also usually organised separately.

From the nursing point of view, then, each of the wards acted in most respects as a 'self-contained unit', communicating up the hierarchy to those above but not particularly along the hierarchy with peers in other wards or units. Appeals for staffing help had to go through the central office and neither Sister or the nurse-in-charge could appeal directly to their neighbours. Because each ward Sister and her team were responsible for practice in their area, they were made increasingly accountable as individuals. In dividing wards one from the other, there was little possibility for collective action and, potentially, nurses may have been easier to 'rule'.

Importantly, in complete contrast to the medical staff, nurses mostly related to the ward as an 'isolated' and enclosed domain. On a daily basis their important association was with medical staff rather than with a 'body' of nurses.

The social: geriatric medicine

A consultant geriatrician, and his senior registrar were attached to the unit in a consultative capacity. One or both of these doctors visited twice a week. On their first visit of the week they 'picked up' (the geriatrician's term) all patients over the age of 65. On their second visit they conducted the 'social round' where all elderly patients were presented and discussed with other members of various disciplines.

The inclusion of geriatric medical staff can be understood partly as an effect of historical problems in the hospital, and partly because of changes in the organisation of the NHS. National concerns at the time over value for money and efficiency brought about the introduction of general management into the health services (Strong & Robinson, 1990). Devices which had already emerged to help make the hospital more efficient included the opening of a day case unit and an admissions unit. This meant that several medical wards changed their use so that the remaining wards had to increase the number of times per week that they had beds available for admitting acutely ill patients.

While there were no formal throughput targets set at this time, the new arrangements had the effect of making it imperative that each medical ward got patients through the beds faster than before. However, each medical ward still took any adult patient of any age admitted to the hospital with a medical condition.

The patients

One of the most prominent types of patient who blocked beds were older patients. In this way, older people had been constituted as a target to be managed by people with specialist knowledge, geriatricians, drawing on a relatively recent social technology, geriatric assessment.

The 20 people around whom this study focused were all over the age of 75. As stated in the introduction this group of patients constituted a special case for nursing assessment. They were all suffering from a multitude of troubles which brought them to Accident and Emergency (A&E).

Mrs Violet, Mrs Adamson, Mr Blakely and Mrs Gardner had terrible pains in their chests. Many of the patients also had trouble with their hearts not beating hard enough or fast enough, or too fast or irregularly – and this gave them trouble breathing and caused swelling in their legs. Major Stevenson and Mr Malone had infections and were highly feverish, with rigors and weakness. Mr Black and Mr Donald had suffered strokes which interfered with them thinking clearly, talking, walking or doing any of the usual things they did. Some had been generally unwell for several days, like

Mrs Appleton, and had collapsed in the street, in a shop or at home and had vague symptoms, such as problems with passing water. Mrs Marsh had inhaled a pea and suffered a 'frightening', prolonged attack of choking and subsequent severe breathlessness. She also had trouble with swollen ankles and apparently her heart was not beating properly.

Some of these elderly people had several problems. Mrs Best had blood coming from an ulcer in the wall of her stomach which gave her black diarrhoea and made her sick, and this was on top of a colostomy and severe arthritis which made her joints deformed so she walked with a stick. Mrs Best was so stiff she could hardly get up in the morning or comb her hair, or cut up her food without taking her arthritis tablets, which were probably the cause of the ulcer in her stomach. Mrs Menzies had an open tumour in her breast, which she had concealed for eight years. Her cancer had spread in her body so that she had water in her abdomen which could find no way out because her heart was failing. She had diarrhoea and could not hold her urine or her stools. Mrs Weston, who was 88, had been run over by a car, had broken a bone in her arm and her pelvis, and was covered with swelling and bruises. The shock had apparently made her bleed from her stomach.

Three of the patients, Miss Hepburn, Mr Donald and Mr MacIntosh, lived on their own and had collapsed and lain all night on the floor. Two of these people, Miss Hepburn and Mr MacIntosh, were in their late eighties and, when put in the hospital, nobody knew what was wrong or was sure if they could think clearly enough to look after themselves any more at home, even with lots of support. Both were not discharged and stayed in hospital before being placed elsewhere. One man, Mr Wallace, who was 90, was severely disabled with Parkinson's disease. He had collapsed at home and was semi-conscious. He was thought to have had a heart attack and pneumonia and he died a few days later.

All the patients had families. Some had busy and active social lives. Some lived on their own but had children or close relatives, as well as neighbours, district nurses, home helps and other support in their lives. Being at home for all the people I talked to was about networking. These social networks were based around other people but also included 'shared' activities, such as cooking, talking, shopping, visiting, sharing meals (one woman's granddaughter came every day from school for her lunch), games, television (particularly for news), the telephone, newspapers, crosswords, books, sewing, knitting, sport, religion and music. As Mrs Best said, 'keeping young is about staying in touch, staying interested'.

Most of the people I talked to had lives rich with the present as well as the past. They drew on culturally available materials to perform an identity which helped differentiate them and qualify their belonging to one category of person rather than another, whether it be concerned and responsible husband, attractive woman or caring mother. In particular, many of the older people I talked to emphasised that they were engaged in active, caring and productive relationships. However, they also appeared to be concerned about the balance of these relationships, by what they called dependency, and expressed fear at the idea of being any more dependent than they were. Many of them therefore considered that interdependence and reciprocity were important to their identity. Some said that they would rather be dead or put in a home than be a burden to others. For example, here is an extract from Mr Donald's interview. I had just asked him how he felt about the future:

> **Mr Donald:** As far as I'm concerned I've felt for over a year that I should be dead, ready laid, right, no regrets, dead! I want to die, I want to die, I want to die!
>
> **JL:** Is that how you're feeling?
>
> **Mr Donald:** That's how I've felt for over a year: I want to die, because I've nothing to live for. I'm a man who's never owed other people and I'm having to depend on other people to look after me and I don't want that. I'd rather be dead. See?
>
> **JL:** Really?
>
> **Mr Donald:** But as far as I'm concerned, when I get to have my (recovery?/discharge?) I'll make the best of it and go home and see how things go. So far, but oh, I would just love something to happen so that I could just slip away and be finished with it all.

In his account Mr Donald is presenting himself as someone who is not normally dependent: he was a man who never owed anybody. But he does not leave the matter there, he would lose face as miserable and ungrateful. He may write himself off, but he does not want others to do so. He offers another face: he's resigned to make the best of a bad job and just 'see how things go'.

Dependency and becoming a burden were common characteristics in many of the patients' discourses, which is relevant to how some older people conduct themselves. This theme revolves around the notion that 'the essence of meaning and fulfilment in later life (the opposite of loneliness and anomie) lies in belonging and participating in family, community, peer groups, reference groups, and other forms of group life' (Peterson, 1985, p. 10).

Family

Access by families to patients is controlled in the hospital. As with all 'visitors' they are only allowed in at visiting times which lasted for two and half hours each day.

During the study it was noticed that family did work in the ward. They delivered information about their relative to and from staff. The nursing staff's appreciation of family was ambivalent: on the one hand staff worked to make sense of the relationship of the family to the patient, in terms of the support they were prepared to give, so family was seen both as a source of information and a source of support for discharge. Where support from the family was forthcoming the relatives were seen to be 'good'. But they were also regarded as a 'nuisance' when it came to wanting information because they were seen as interrupting the work of the ward. This may have been related to the difficulties that some nursing staff expressed about being kept up-to-date with information from doctors. Some nursing staff stated that they did not always have information about overall medical plans for patients or their diagnoses, and one nurse told me that she found it 'undermining' when families pressed for information which was unforthcoming from the doctors.

Where a patient was seen to be dying, staff regarded the family as included in their domain of care: the family became needy and nurses were there to help them in their need. Dying was constituted partly through a termination of treatment, where 'nature is allowed to take its course'. Under these circumstances, the family was given more open access to be with the dying patient. This relies, of course, on staff realising that 'nature is taking its course' and that a patient is indeed dying. The staff have to 'change gear' and alter their mode of activity. Changing gear depends upon staff refiguring a patient's identity, from being seen as someone who is being treated to someone who is dying. During the study one patient died before staff had realised that she was dying and family were not included until after the event. Processes of recategorising patients are very complex, and will be returned to as central to how nurses conduct ward life.

For those patients who had been in hospital a long time the family were also allowed in at irregular times to take patients out and provide what one nurse described as a 'social' life, which the nurses said they could not provide. Some of the nurses described how the ward had become 'home' for these patients. This made it different; this meant that a social life was something the patients needed.

Differentiating patients

Categories are the most basic form of hospital organisation. The hospital dealt in 'beds', 'admissions' and 'discharges'. All these expressions were in the day-to-day talk of staff. But such categories are metonymic, where a part of a system or process stands for the whole (Osterwalder, 1978). For example, the expression 'bed' signifies many resources: a space available to place someone in, the hospital's facilities, expertise, nurses, drinks, machines, cleaning, research, drugs, shelter, food, work.

On the other hand the use of the term 'bed' is also metaphoric: it helps to signify movement, movement through the hospital, the flow. Critically, to gain access to a bed, a person has to be categorised appropriately. The two routes into the hospital to gain access to a bed were either via out-patients or via A&E, with or without a GP referral. Getting access to a bed through either of these routes meant the person had to be constituted in some way as an 'admission'. This involved staff in processes of 'naming'.

The study concentrated on elderly people who had little or no warning that they would soon find themselves in hospital. All the patients in the study were admitted via A&E. Once through A&E they became an 'admission', designated an 'acute' or an 'emergency' admission. That is, to gain access to a bed, they were considered by A&E staff to belong to an appropriate category. From documentary evidence this process could take up to five hours. This seems to indicate that processes of admission were complex and that people arriving at A&E, older people at least, were not admitted lightly. How was this admission process accomplished?

Accessing a medical bed

The person presenting at A&E to be admitted to an 'acute medical ward' had to be assessed by the medical staff to be a medical admission, rather than any other type of admission. They had to be given a differential diagnosis, even if this was only provisional, such as 'possible myocardial infarction (heart attack)'. On their arrival, people presenting to A&E were seen by the doctor on duty* and then if he/she deemed it appropriate they were referred to the 'medical registrar' for a second opinion. It would then be up to the medical registrar to decide if the person would be admitted to a medical ward (or the cardiac care unit), or whether the patient would be more appropriately sent home or referred to another speciality for their opinion.

In this way the person was not simply constituted as an admission in A&E but was assessed to be a specific type of admission – he or she was 'named' according to a code and this naming allowed them to be assigned a place within the hospital. This, in turn, led to their geographical placement in a bed in a specific ward.

---

* Recently another layer has been added to the process of gaining a bed: nurse triage. In some A&E units the first contact the patient has with the clinical staff is a triage nurse. He or she ranks patients in order of priority or relays them elsewhere. The amount of discretion a triage nurse has varies considerably across the country and from Trust to Trust.

The ways in which the hospital was organised in relation to the allo-cation of the main resource, the 'beds', depended upon naming and placing of people as patients according to not just medical speciality, but also their translation into hospital discourse. The person became named as an entity which could be organised: an 'acute medical admission' can be placed within an acute medical ward. These processes can be considered to be methods of categorisation which require staff to use 'systems of dis-tinction' (Deetz, 1992). These distinctions are not necessarily self-evident, although they may have the appearance of being taken for granted. For an ethnographer, it is how these distinctions are made up and deployed which require close examination. As will be seen, differentiating patients does not rest upon medical discursive practices alone, although it is important for staff to maintain an appearance that this is the case.

It is important, then, to recognise that patients arrive on the wards 'prefigured'. Once on the ward this 'figuring' process continues from there. But there are other aspects of the hospital admission process which affected how ward staff categorised and recategorised patients. The aspect which I want to focus on concerns what I have referred to earlier as 'the flow'. An emphasis on beds and bed availability affects ward staff's assessments of patients and the way in which patients are put into one category (say, acute medical) rather than another (say, chronically medical).

Waiting

The waiting system is an organising device which helps maintain the ebb and flow of patients through beds. Changes to this waiting system meant that time became more pressing in a number of ways and this affected the way in which staff worked.

Every fourth day one of the consultants on the unit was responsible for admitting patients with a 'medical diagnosis' from A&E and for taking patients ready for transfer from CCU. Prior to the commencement of the study each ward had to wait seven days for this to happen. This change in organisational arrangements was due to more widespread changes in hospital use which were aimed at making the hospital more efficient. In practice, the increase in the number of days that each ward had to be 'on take' meant that there was a considerable reduction in the time staff had to 'turn patients around' from admission to discharge. This organisational change had a profound effect on staff's practices. First, it focused staff on a patient's potential for discharge *from the moment of their admission* to the wards. Second, it reinforced specialisation and narrowed the scope for what needs or troubles were included as appropriate to an acute care context.

Staff therefore (partly) organised their days and their relationships with each other around their waiting days. They timed discharges, not necessarily because the patient needed to be in hospital still, but to coincide with their waiting day, to ensure that they had beds available to take new admissions. As stated earlier, the nursing hierarchy did not audit care, but did stress the delivery of empty beds as an indication of competence. Key locations for these processes were the ward round and the social round. The 'waiting' consultant did a ward round with his medical staff and the nurse-in-charge of the admissions unit at 8am on 'Post Waiting Day' on the admissions ward. Patients requiring further care were then transferred on to the waiting ward sometime during the morning. The waiting ward nursing staff had no control over who was admitted to their ward and they were not represented in A&E or on the Post Waiting Day ward round on the admissions ward.

Although there were no critical pathways or clinical guidelines in place at the time of the study, the waiting system had the effect of helping ensure that staff were aware of how long patients were taking to get better. This in turn led to semi-formal benchmarks and protocols over how a patient should have progressed given their time in hospital and their diagnosis.

In order to be able to take patients from A&E, CCU and from the admissions ward, the waiting ward had to make beds available on both waiting day and the day subsequent to waiting day. This means that staff arranged for patients to be discharged on these days – discharges were 'staggered' by the nurses over the two days so that beds became available at the right time and were not 'taken' by other wards. Sometimes this meant that discharges were planned to coincide with the need to have beds available, not just with the cessation of a patient's need for care.

The effects of focusing nurses on a patient's future (as a discharge) potentially lead to difficulties over focusing attention on a patient's *current* state. This in turn reinforces something endemic to hospital care: a difficulty with attending to the patient as an experiencing and present subject. These admissions and discharge arrangements have the potential then to 'industrialise' hospital care, reducing the patient to an object to be processed, and of cementing nurses' relationships with patients as one of instrumentalism. An organisational agenda which demands greater differentiation is therefore potentially incompatible with the ethos central to nursing discourse (Chapter 1) that nurses should be concerned with all aspects of a patient's health. Nurses are in danger of being given an endless ethical dilemma. The question that arises is how do nurses square this dilemma?

Appropriate patients

Nurses square their dilemma by differentiating need, and the practices required to meet these needs, into either social or medical. The complex arrangements for the admission of patients to the 'main' hospital have deep meanings for nurses. They are associated with making sure the right sorts of patients get admitted to the right kinds of beds. The right sorts of patients are not just those with interesting diseases or who need a lot of care, rather they are those patients who have the potential for speedy recovery. Under these conditions to be a good or a 'first class patient' a patient must have a condition which may be considered *initially* as acute, but which has the potential for resolution so that he or she can be returned *in good time* to a category of patient which is dischargable. In other words, a patient's condition must be acute, serious and resolvable. Only in this way can a patient's career through the hospital satisfy the demand for speed as well as demonstrable outcomes.

That a patient's appropriateness had come to matter in this particular sense is exemplified by a conversation I had with several qualified nurses on Ward 1 soon after commencing the study. I asked Sister what she thought the rationale was behind the opening of the admissions ward (until recently patients were admitted onto the main wards during the night as well as during the day). She and two of the staff nurses were at the nurses' station:

Sister: It's to stop the wards being disturbed at night.
Senior staff nurse: It's also so that some patients can be discharged straight home if necessary. A lot of patients are geriatric and should never get to the medical wards.
Sister: They're admitted because they've fallen at home and they need mobilising and rehabilitation, physiotherapy and occupational therapy. But they're admitted here and they're here for weeks. They don't have any medical problems.
JL: So what is a 'geriatric' patient?
Sister: Elderly.
Senior staff nurse: Frail, old, gone off their legs a bit.
Staff nurse (who had been listening while at the drug trolley): Ward 10 [the geriatric assessment ward in the hospital] is always half empty and they're admitted here because they won't take acute admissions to the ward there, only referrals.

The nurses indicate in this conversation that there are inappropriately placed people in their ward. The nurses assert that geriatric patients require different care from people with 'medical problems'. To do this the nurses are putting in play and playing upon a set of distinctions: geriatrics have special 'needs' which can be met through specific skills and facilities, such as 'mobilising and rehabilitation, physiotherapy and occupational therapy'. These skills and facilities and the needs they are designed to meet are different from those of an acute medical ward.

Central to the way the hospital was organised, then, was this concept of appropriateness constituted through systems of distinction. But the naming was taken by the nurses to be already 'given' to some extent – in the conversation it was as if a patient was revealed as falling into a category which was or was not appropriate. A person was identified and named as a patient who had 'medical problems' rather than as a 'geriatric', 'gone off their legs', 'frail, old'. Nurses thus engaged in systems of distinction which differentiated patients as appropriate or not.

Inappropriate patients and the social

In the following extract the same staff nurse and Sister go on to talk about a patient who is 'long-term'. The distinctions they make help to illustrate how they are figuring what constitutes appropriateness and inappropriateness.

> **Sister:** Take Jessie. She came to us as a purely social admission. She'd fallen at home and is incontinent. She had turned against her home help, refused to answer the door to let her in. She didn't become 91 over night, she's been old for a long time. She had been going downhill and she's been here ever since. She didn't have any medical problems. What is the GP doing, is what I would like to know. She should have been on the long-term waiting list and assessed by the GP and admitted there, not here.
> **JL:** So why did she come in?
> **Sister:** She had fallen. She is incontinent.

At some level Sister is justifying that the flow through the bed has been interrupted. Jessie is stuck on the ward, is long-term, and Sister has a 'blocked bed'. In order to provide a justification Sister assembles a number of matters to support her case: she devolves blame onto others (the patient and the GP) and she marks out her territory. To justify the state of affairs, Sister enrols a distinction to make her story: the patient is a 'purely social admission'.

Now the interesting aspect here is how having medical problems is different from being geriatric or being 'social'. Incontinence and falls change their character depending on the context in which they are viewed, and the Sister assembles various facts to provide that context. Indeed, the details of Jessie's context, the aspects of her social and medical history which are put into play by the Sister, change the nature of her needs so that Jessie is characterised as having social, rather than medical, needs. This then classifies Jessie as inappropriate.

Here follows the final part of the exchange:

JL: What about the stroke? [Jessie's 'diagnosis' at report was cerebro-vascular accident]
Staff nurse: Oh, she had that after she came in. She's gone down-hill. She used to walk with a zimmer and dress and wash herself. That's how she managed at home. Now she needs long term care.
Sister: She is purely a social problem.
JL: So why did she fall ?
Staff nurse: She had gone off her legs a bit, frail, you know, old and frail.

Even though Jessie has had a stroke she is still considered to be a 'social problem', not a medical one. As such she is not considered appropriate to an acute medical ward.

So how is this possible? Sister and the staff nurse drew upon culturally available ground to support their case in figuring Jessie as 'not medical'. This was done by bringing into play the matter of time: 'She had not become 91 overnight, she's been old for a long time', 'She's been going down hill', 'She needs long term care'. Being old over time is different from being ill and being medical. Sister enrolled the cultural notion that illness in old age at some point becomes something which is natural and to be expected. Illness and pathology therefore become non-medical as they become the natural consequence of biological decline. At this point the needs arising from such illness become social needs, which are different from those needs which are the responsibility of the acute health services. The nurses thus partially disposed of their dilemma through a distinction between their work in an acute medical domain and other kinds of work, which are social, not medical. They disposed of their sense of responsibility for Jessie's needs by characterising them again as social, not medical. In doing this they formed limits to acute medicine and, at the same time, they helped recompose the quality of first class medicine as well as construct their own identities.

The reality of nursing

The nurses at Royal University Hospital did not generally give a sense of doubting that what they were doing was 'right'. Although the nurses told me that it seemed that 'they [the hospital and nursing administration] were only interested in beds', they showed almost no signs of resisting. In the following extract a staff nurse articulates the tension that is created by pressure on beds and time, but she also indicates how that tension is resolved. She gives a picture of what her priorities were at the time and how she had to act to fulfil them. In her representation of herself and how the ward was organised, she treads a fine line between ambivalence toward her role and exhibiting a kind of streetwise attitude to nursing practice:

> **Staff nurse:** It's difficult when you're in charge because you end up with ... [pause]. You can only talk to people you feel particularly need to be spoken to, and your assessment of that might not be quite right. You might not pick up on the people that do need to sit and chat to somebody, who can answer their questions and what have you. It's something I try to do but it's sometimes difficult. It has been recently to find the time. Maybe we have false priorities – we think that everybody wants to be washed, maybe that's not the case, maybe some people don't want to be bothered about being washed. You know, we think we've got to do that!

The staff nurse indicated that patients are nursed to a great extent according to the routine. During the interview she revealed that she believed at one level that it was only through working with patients, getting to know them and talking with them that she could really understand their needs. However, as a staff nurse, she could not always achieve this kind of contact. Continuing the conversation, she stated that it was the students who had close relationships with patients and she felt her priorities had gradually changed:

> **Staff nurse:** You're either directly or indirectly responsible for what's going on. When you start off you say 'well, I would want to do what the patient would want me to do'. You know, if the patient wants me to sit and blether for half an hour, I would want to sit and blether with them, but in reality, within the constraints of the ward, the ward routine and the set routine and what other people are expecting of you, need from you ...
> **JL:** Other people being?
> **Staff nurse:** Other patients, medical staff, other learners, and what have you. You tend to end up in a routine and you know, you get somebody up, you give somebody their breakfast, you make somebody's bed, and then you help them to wash, you know, whatever. Wash them whatever it is.

The staff nurse located the change in herself to her adaptation to what she called 'reality'. 'Reality' was constituted by the 'constraints of the ward', 'the ward routine', and 'what other people expect/need from you'.

'Reality' was not directly constituted by patients' needs. Below she shows how she saw her adaptation to 'reality' as a part of her 'socialisation'.

> **Staff nurse:** I think you gradually become socialised into the system and nursing. You know, nursing's a routine.
> **JL:** To get the routine through is your priority?
> **Staff nurse:** To a certain extent it is, and sometimes I feel very guilty about that and I think 'that's ridiculous, that's terrible', and then at other times I think 'but we are, this is an acute hospital and you have got to be in a state of readiness, for an emergency, or for a turn of events'.

For this nurse prioritising the routine was related to what she believed to be the nature and purpose of the hospital. She articulated what was evident in nurses' practices: a fundamental expectation that the ward staff will ensure that beds are available when it is their turn, and to be in a state of readiness to deal with emergencies as they arise. What this staff nurse knows is that to be the nurse-in-charge she has to get through the routine. For her this is legitimated by what she believes to be the nature and purpose of her work in the acute hospital. She indicates that this frequently conflicted with what patients wanted or needed and this left her with feelings of 'guilt' and 'frustration'. However, she was later able to rationalise her actions to some extent by saying that the patients themselves need routine and quickly adapt to it.

The staff nurse may have been attempting, in some of her comments, to present a 'nurse' whom she thought would be more acceptable to me, the researcher, than the nurse I saw at work. I had been observing her at work for close on three months and her report of her self and her priorities was congruent with the impression I had of her as she went about her duties. Her beliefs about her activities and the rationalisations she made exemplified the 'image' she had of herself as someone both *acting on* the world and as someone being *acted upon* by the world ('socialised', the demands of others, the system) in the name of something larger than herself – the need to be ready to cope with the acutely ill by having beds available and by being in a state of readiness.

The conversation with the staff nurse encapsulates the tension which all nurses continuously experience. This tension is created by pressure from the patients already in their care and the pressure (made continuously present in their lives by devices such as waiting day) for them to attend to the mass of absent and faceless (but *ideal*) acute patients potentially thronging for beds. These ideal, acute patients never materialise. Instead, their mythical presence is always held on a future horizon. At the same time, their amorphous shape presses nurses to continuously efface those needs which are extraneous to the work of an acute ward. After all, the staff nurse characterised a patient's need to talk as 'blethering' and in doing this she downgraded it. There is something then which is *insignificant* about needs which are not medical.

Discussion

In evoking the hospital as a 'complex location' this chapter has shown how nurses work to multiple agendas. First, the nurses in the study were employed in an internationally famous UK teaching hospital and their work involved the accomplishment of 'first class medicine'. First class medicine is purely clinical. To be pure, clinical medicine effaces the social and is premised on disciplined and objective knowledge. This is because it is only purely clinical medicine that makes the causes of death, pain and suffering visible. Although the doctors were themselves mostly absent from ward life, the medical agenda was made present in almost all aspects of hospital organisation, from categories of ward and patients, through to the ways in which the ward rounds were conducted.

But 'visualising' disease is not enough. Under the microscope of management, medicine is increasingly being judged by its effects. The second agenda, then, is that the nurses' work involves accomplishing health and social policy. In today's NHS, nurses and doctors are continually faced with delivering a public service to consumers as individuals but at the same time they are charged with getting more medicine to more people. The ways in which the waiting system has been changed help to make this second agenda present in the day-to-day lives of nurses. The pressure on staff over beds has been increased over a period of two years by increasing responsibility for 'waiting' from one day in six to one day in four. By having beds available to take new admissions, the acutely ill have, to some extent, been made to dominate hospital life for both staff and patients. For staff, having beds available on 'waiting day' and the following day is a mark of efficiency and the ability to cope. It is one way that the effectiveness and efficiency of nurses' work are made visible to managers and to themselves.

These two agendas illustrate the tension between managing and care. They could be taken to represent two competing moral discourses: a utilitarian discourse, which demands that more people are treated, and a professional discourse of care for the individual. There is therefore a third agenda which nurses are working to, a professional agenda which stresses nurturing and caring. By examining the nurses' conversation about Jessie it emerged that nurses can partly reconcile these agendas with their own professional requirement to take all of a person's needs into consideration. They do this by distinguishing between two kinds of needs, social and medical. Nurses are also aware of the discrepancy between the professional emphasis on doing what patients say they need, and the demands of caring for more than one person in a service situation. The reality of nursing somehow consists of balancing these agendas.

Specifically then, nurses work in a policy context in which medicine is not unproblematically on tap. Medicine and care are to be distributed as scarce *social* resources. Distribution depends upon criteria and processes of inclusion and exclusion and within this context only some patients will do. The next chapter is concerned with how nurses organise themselves, the wards and patients. It explores how nurses are implicated in accomplishing first class medicine in a world of limited resources and demonstrable outcomes.

Chapter 3
Organising Ward Life

Introduction

As Chapter 2 indicated, ward life is organised. But who does this work? What influences how ward life is organised? Competing contenders are patients' needs, doctors' orders, managerial objectives, and a nursing discourse that stresses the holistic care of patients as individuals. However, each of these contenders is itself open to differences in interpretation.

Many organisational devices are designed to make ward life predictable, standardised and controllable. Traditional methods of regulation include explicit rules, like those expressed in hospital procedures and policies. But in the 1980s and 1990s there were shifts to more diverse methods of regulation, which depended upon staff regulating themselves. These more recent forms of regulation include 'social' technologies, like the nursing process, as well as devices like waiting days, discussed in the previous chapter. Critically, the organisation of ward life depends upon nurses working with, and being worked by, these different forms of regulation.

This chapter presents material that shows how nurses order ward life through nursing handovers, ward routines and the use of space and time. The chapter examines each of these practices in turn in order to illustrate how ward life is something which nurses *produce*. The main point is that the work of balancing the different agendas discussed in Chapter 2 engages nurses in practices of inclusion and exclusion through which patients, nurses and types of work become differentiated and hierarchised. Appendix 5 contains a brief guide to ward organisation and the organisation of labour at the Royal University Hospital.

Handovers: the division of labour and the labour of division

In the nursing handover two critical aspects of organisation emerge. First, at the handover work is allocated between different levels and types of nurse. This division of labour shows how types of work, including speaking about patients, are both differentiated and hierarchised. For example, only qualified nurses are permitted to speak at the handover. Second, the handover also constitutes 'a labour of division' (see Hetherington & Munro, 1997), in that the handover relays to nurses not just what aspects of the patients and nursing work have more significance than others, but *how significance is accomplished.*

Nursing handovers take place at each change of shift, either at the nurses' station or in Sister's office. The nurse handing over has the nursing 'Kardex' in front of her, the metal folder containing all the nursing records, including the nurses' copy of the accident and emergency admission document (called the 'pink slip'). She goes through written records of each patient in sequence as they are situated around the ward. The other nurses sit opposite her, making notes in their personal note books or on scraps of paper.

The nurse handing over will either hand over or report to nurses on her own shift (the early handover) or she will hand over to nurses on the next shift (the midday and the late to night staff handover). The handover nurse is the nurse in charge of the shift and, as such, is the most senior nurse on duty for that shift (except for the night shift where the staff nurse and the state-enrolled nurse take it in turns to hand over to the day shift). The late to night staff handovers and the night staff to early shift handovers last about ten to fifteen minutes in total. The early staff handovers last about twenty minutes to half an hour. The midday handover lasts from half an hour to three-quarters of an hour. This in when most information about patients is relayed.

The person handing over is always a qualified nurse. The nurse doing the handover sometimes reads from the 'Kardexes' or the 'pink slip' and sometimes speaks without reading but looking directly at the nurses grouped in front of her. One aspect of the handover is the allocation of work. On the early shift nurses are given 'bays' of patients to look after, while the late shift nurses are given half the ward to look after. Usually, the bays are allocated to a pair of nurses. Sometimes specific patients are mentioned and allocated to a specific nurse. Where a patient is being nursed in a cubicle and is very ill this is called 'specialing' a patient, and usually this would be a nurse's only responsibility for a shift. Specific allocation might simply entail a nurse being given particular responsibility for a patient and asked to carry out a certain aspect of care, for example, when someone is very ill and is 'for all two-hourly care', or needs rehydrating and is 'on two-hourly fluids', or 'on observations' which are more frequent than at the routine times, such as two-hourly neurological observations. In these ways the division of labour is organised, not in a fixed allocation system but in ways which are reflexive to skill mix and the level of dependency of patients as assessed by the nurses in charge.

The handover is routinised. The handover nurse gives particular details of the patient (e.g. name, age, diagnosis, relevant medical problems), then may go on to describe their current condition or give some account of what had happened during the shift in terms of observations, any investigations undertaken, medications given or specific (as opposed to routine) nursing care. She may then give instructions for nursing care, observations, medications or investigations for the next shift. The extent of the handover material and length of time spent on a patient varies from a few seconds to five minutes. The most time is spent on new patients, patients with apparently complicated problems or very ill patients. Long-term patients and patients close to discharge typically have short handover times.

Nursing handovers are usually one-way communication channels for information and instruction to go down, along or up the hierarchy. The handover nurse tells the others about patients and there is not usually any conversation or turn-taking. In this way the handovers are not usually forums for discussion about patients in terms either of what had been noticed about them, what inferences can be drawn or what care patients might require in response to any particular problem. Similarly they are not usually spaces for speculation or explanation about conditions, aspects of nursing care, consequences of illness or patients' meanings, except in unusual circumstances.

The handovers change over time. The handovers closest to the admission of the patient focus on recording and making sense of a patient's observed condition in relation to their possible medical condition. Subsequently handovers focus more on mobilising patients. Sometimes nurses pass on details about a patient's home life and mental state right at the beginning of their admission. This is unusual and often signifies that these aspects of a patient are under suspicion.

The handovers make certain aspects of the patient's behaviour or responses significant. They are to be remarked upon and instruct nurses what to look out for. Instruction in the main is implicit not explicit – not only are the nurses giving an account of what they have noticed and done, they are passing on what others can attend to and do. Signification in this way is circulated through processes of iteration. For example, when presenting a patient with a suspected heart attack, a staff nurse might mention what she has been observing during her shift (such as chest pain, nausea, bradycardia) and summarise the patient's condition (he's fine, comfortable, no chest pain). In doing this she implies, rather than instructs, what the nurses on the next shift should themselves attend to (chest pain, nausea, bradycardia). In this way the handovers are like a relay.

At handovers nurses only reflect at length upon those aspects of 'care' which are an anomaly. Care which is anomalous is care which is extraneous to ward routines, such as the administration of special medicines, specific observations, or the use of unusual apparatus, such as heparin pumps.

References to 'nursing care' are also typically implicit, either carried in the diagnosis and condition of the patient or very brief, and consist mainly of short references to global terms such as 'bed rest' or 'self-caring'. In the absence of overt instructions about nursing care the nurses have interpretative work to do; they are left to translate the information given them at handover into both an understanding of a patient's condition and also into specific nursing care. Where there are care plans there is less onus on the nurse, but the care plans are often prepared at the beginning of a patient's stay and do not get updated or lack detail as to basic nursing issues. Also note that the patient's comfort is not the touchstone of nursing activity. This distinction is important – the significance of a patient's troubles almost never derives from a patient-centred perspective. Even chest pain takes its importance from being the sign of an unstable heart rather than as something which is causing the patient pain and fear. This situation arises not because the nurses are heartless but because of the problem of visibility. Patients' feelings and experiences are simply not a strong ground – they are personal, not clinical, matters.

Handovers are discursive when there are things which the nurses have observed about a patient which cannot be expressed routinely. This happens when the nurses' observations of a patient do not fit with what is already known, or where aspects of a patient's condition have the potential to impede their progress and thereby block the flow through the beds. Thus, discontinuities, anomalies, recession or lack of progress can all occasion a more discursive type of nursing handover.

Handing over Mrs Appleton

The following extract exemplifies several of the findings about handovers referred to above:

> **Handover staff nurse** [to the late shift]: Then you have Mrs Wendy Appleton, an 81-year-old lady who came in on the 10th with chest pain. She's for exclusion of MI [myocardial infarction or heart attack] and treatment of a UTI [urinary tract infection]. She had a four day history of general malaise. But yesterday morning she just went out – she was in her bed, head slumped down. She had a strong regular pulse and her B/P was okay [the phone rings and the handover staff nurse answers it. The call finishes after a few minutes.] Uh ... [turns back to Kardex] ... she was unconscious for about three minutes. It resolved itself, she just

gradually came round. An hour later the same thing happened again and it resolved itself. She's twitching all the time – when she holds your hand she sort of grabs it and can't let go. She's on a chart for recording these episodes – like this – if she's drowsy or unconscious or anything.

Senior staff nurse [to late shift nurses]: You had better check her obs [observations] as well at the time.

Handover staff nurse: She was OK last night. Then this morning she felt a bit odd – she didn't tell us until afterwards – but she felt dizzy.

Senior staff nurse [has been looking over at the patient who is lying in the bed next to the nurses' station with cot-sides up]: Has she got a 24-hour tape[1] on?

Handover staff nurse: Yes.

Senior staff nurse: She's in bed. Is she to be kept in bed?

Handover staff nurse: Well, yes. When she sits up she ... it happened yesterday after she'd been sat up for her breakfast and after the doctor took her blood.

Senior staff nurse: We'd better sit her up then, if she's got the 24-hour tape on. Did they say she isn't to sit up?

Handover staff nurse: Er ... no, I don't know. She was incontinent of urine yesterday. We didn't observe it but we think it may have been one of these episodes.

Senior staff nurse [to the late shift nurses]: Before you sit her up, do her erect and supine blood pressure[2], then sit her up.

The handover staff nurse has been in charge on the morning shift. At handover the staff nurse tells the others about what she has seen and makes it clear that what she has seen does not yet add up, or make medical sense. The handover illustrates how, where there is an ambiguity in the patient's symptoms given what is already known about the patient, there is extra conversation and a break in the usual routine. The handover nurse is also doing something more – she is relaying the idea that an important aspect of nurses' work is to help make sense of patients as patients. I want to call this work 'figuring' patients.

To make medical sense the nurses bring into play different kinds of materials. The staff nurse and the senior staff nurse assemble many different materials to 'figure' Mrs Appleton: her age, her name, her history, her diagnosis, the observation of her period of unconsciousness, the doctor's conduct and orders. Instructions as to how she is to be nursed are implicit in the handover and in the exchange between the two staff nurses, apart from those pertaining to the 24-hour tape. How the patient may feel is not explored. The handover also tells the nurses that there are important protocols to be followed (bed rest during the initial admission period), but that these can be mediated to facilitate medical diagnosis. Critically, what is being circulated is that the important aspect about this patient is the observation of her 'episodes'.

Although Mrs Appleton is being figured through medico-technical representations of her body, she is also being put in a context, constructed through the observation of her behaviour: 'She's twitching all the time – when she holds your hand she sort of grabs it and can't let go'. Therefore, while little is said explicitly about how Mrs Appleton feels, the staff nurse puts into play an observation which could reframe other aspects of her 'case': she twitches and grabs and cannot let go.

So the nurses observe patients' behaviour to figure them as persons. It is this supplementary work which provides the context in which a patient's troubles can be interpreted and named. In this particular case, Mrs Appleton's behaviour may be being read as indicative of psychological problems, thus making available a different ground upon which to explain her blackouts – she may be anxious, rather than medically sick.

In this handover the hierarchical division of labour becomes explicit. At handovers the qualified nurses are the ones who speak about patients. Students are silent. They do not have permission to speak, just as they do not have permission to write care plans. This particular handover illustrates how the hierarchy over permission to speak is maintained. In this particular instance the nurse handing over is a recently qualified staff nurse and the receiving staff nurse is the senior staff nurse. The handover becomes an occasion for a call to account and goes into an explicitly instructive mode. The exchange between the two staff nurses helps relay to junior nurses that nurses are accountable for what they do, but that the sources of permission which nurses rely upon to know how to proceed are complex. Critically, it seems that doctors' orders can over-ride usual protocols in certain circumstances.

The effects of the nursing handover in helping to produce hierarchies and systems of difference are further enhanced through the ways in which nursing work is delegated and organised. These matters are now examined in relation to ward routines.

The placing of patients

The placing of patients in the wards also reflected the continuous labour by which nurses differentiated and hierarchised patients, types of work and types of nurse.

Each ward in the hospital in the study had four bays, two side rooms and a side ward. Each of these spaces emerges as having a particular character and this was connected to the ways in which patients' needs, and the skills and facilities required to meet these needs, were classified in the unit.

The qualified nurses in the study all stated that nurses were allocated to the bays according to their level of skill and experience. Junior and auxiliary nurses were given bay 1, the side wards and bay 4 to look after and were supervised by a qualified nurse whenever possible. Bays 2 and 3, especially 3, were allocated to a qualified or senior student nurse or a qualified nurse with a junior student nurse. Bays 2 and 3 were where the new admissions and the 'acute patients' were placed. Very sick patients who were ' being treated' were also placed in these bays, while, according to the Sisters and staff nurses, very sick patients who were 'dying' and who were not being treated were placed in the side rooms. 'Long-term' patients waiting to be re-placed elsewhere, as well as a few convalescent patients and rehabilitation patients, were put in bay 4. Many of the patients in bay 4 were disabled but were no longer considered to be 'medically' ill. They were not called 'medical' patients but were categorised as other types of patients: 'dependent', 'geriatric', 'social', 'demented' or 'disabled'.

Patients for convalescence were placed in bay 1 and the side ward, while rehabilitation patients were placed in bays 1, 2 and 4. This included some stroke patients.

Staff in both wards talked about 'our bay 4' as being not 'too bad' or 'being heavy'. In Ward 1, nurses often referred to 'the bay 4 ladies' and one of the middle-grade doctors referred to bay 4 on the female ward as the 'cabbage patch'. Bay 4 patients were thus grouped, they were not thought of as individuals.

From the nurses' accounts it appears that the distribution of patients in the different bays depended upon the facilities available in each bay and on the amount of observation a patient needed. I asked one of the Sisters to talk about how she arranged the ward.

> **JL:** So when you're allocating nurses to patients in the morning, how would you decide which nurses are going to work with which patients?
> **Sister:** It depends whether I've got trained nurses on or student nurses on. I tend to allocate. I take the patient priority of care so I allocate the most senior people to look after the sickest patients who need specific nursing care.
> **JL:** The most ill. And then you work your way down?
> **Sister:** I work my way down the off-duty [the off-duty goes down in terms of hierarchy, with Sister at the top]. I don't like to allocate two junior students to work on a bay so I try to have a senior nurse and a junior nurse working together, or a senior nurse and an auxiliary nurse working together so that they are supervised.

Sister accounts for her allocation of nurses to patients in terms of 'patient priority of care'. The most 'senior people' ... 'look after the sickest patients' and those who need 'specific nursing care'. Junior nurses are allocated to look after less ill patients, but are supervised. From the rest of the interview (below) it can be seen that Sister figures 'sickest' around two concepts: the observation of patients and what she refers to as 'high-dependency' nursing.

Sister: I have the illest patients in bays 2 and 3, high-dependency nursing in bays 2 and 3.

JL: And why is that, what's your idea?

Sister: Because they're near the station. I think they're near the centre of the ward so they're near the station. You know, there's always people around the station. They can be observed, particularly overnight. That's an excellent place for them to be so they can be observed from the nursing station.

JL: And what about the rest of them?

Sister: The side wards are really just for the convalescing patients or for waiting list patients in for trial drugs or endoscopies, or that's what I use the four-bedded room for. I like to keep the side cubicle for terminally ill patients. Often they are very high-dependency nursing as well, but it's a nice room to keep for the relatives and for the patient. Nice quiet room. Other than that, self-caring patients go into there.

JL: So you use it for the terminal care patients because ... ?

Sister: Obviously we're not going to be actively resuscitating them.

JL: Right.

Sister: And they don't have to be so closely observed for that, although they are high-dependency nursing.

JL: Right, you mean they need a lot of ... ?

Sister: They need a lot of nursing care.

JL: That's interesting. When you say 'high dependency' what sort of things are you thinking of in their care? Although I know you're not observing them like ...

Sister: You're not observing them but you're caring for them, full mouth care, eye care, turning, catheter care normally, perhaps care of an infusion pump. Really, all types of nursing care.

JL: Right. And you also have the relatives.

Sister: The relatives – you've got all the communications with the relatives, and you must spend a long time with these relatives, to be supportive.

JL: Okay, and then you've got bay 4, who do you tend to put there?

Sister: Sorry, I've got bay 1 where I put convalescents, patients who are getting better. Bay 4 is normally used for long-term patients probably because there's no oxygen and suction down there, which is as good a reason as any. Some of my long-term patients if in good [condition] – I wouldn't nurse them down in bay 4.

JL: Why is that?
Sister: Because I would want them to have the stimulation of other patients, of seeing people coming in and out the ward. I would tend to nurse them in bay 1. Patients like Larry.
JL: Like Larry, yes. Because I remember when I first came you were just moving him.
Sister: Moving him up there for the stimulation really. And he has come on you know, they do get stimulated up there.

To account for what she does Sister constructs patients according to types such as 'acute' and 'high-dependency'. She also referred to 'acute admissions', 'convalescent', 'rehabilitative', 'waiting list', 'self-caring', 'terminal care' and 'long-term.' But 'long-term' patients could be 'good' so could become a category on their own. For example, 'good strokes' who need 'stimulation' would represent 'good' long-term patients. Sister also indicates that patients can move from one category to another, for example, 'good strokes' moving from long-term to patients who get 'moved up' for 'stimulation' which helps them 'come on'. She configures these typifications around needs: acute and high-dependency patients need observing and may also need oxygen, suction and other specific nursing care. Stroke patients need stimulation, to see people being busy, coming and going. Terminal patients need peace and quiet with their relatives close by and require high-dependency nursing, but observation is not, literally, vital (they are not for resuscitation) so they can be nursed in a cubicle, out of sight but not out of mind. In contrast long-term patients are left at the back of the ward, out of sight and with no specific nursing requirements, and they can be looked after by junior nurses and auxiliaries who are supervised. Sister remarked elsewhere that these are 'heavy' patients.

Her conversation contains metaphors which help signify the critical place of movement in her typologies: 'up the ward', 'coming along'. Further, it signifies an important system of distinction through which patients were not just being categorised, but also classified. There is a constituting of classes being brought into play here. The terminal and the long-term have no movement and can be out of sight. The long-term and strokes are 'heavy'. This is a descriptive term, a metaphor. Being heavy does not constitute them as 'high dependency', it has a different meaning within these settings. They are heavy on the nurses, and often need two to move them about, they may be disabled and need a lot of help, but they are not 'really sick'. Critically they are longer term and they weigh down the wards because they are difficult to move on.

Place signifying care

As well as helping to order the setting, the placing of patients is an organising device in a second sense. It is through the placing of patients that nurses partly know how to care for them.

Nurses seemed to look for particular types of work according to where the patient was in the ward. For example, a very sick patient in the cubicle might indicate a visit at breakfast time, not to sit them up, but to turn them or give them mouth care or just to see how they are. During the study, nurses working to get the breakfasts out in bay 3 kept most patients in bed until after the nursing handover, as these were the patients who had recently been admitted. Thus, at a practical level, the placing of patients, in concert with the ward routines and discursive practices, acted to signify the type of patients nurses were dealing with and from this they could extrapolate the general forms of care the patient should be given. The places in which patients were situated helped remind and reinforce the types of care that they might require. Rarely, mistakes were made. For example, Mrs Adamson was very unwell on admission. She had been admitted the previous evening with a query heart attack but there were no spaces left in bay 3 and she had been put into bay 2. This may have signified to the nurses that she was not 'that' ill so that they sat her up for breakfast. Sister remarked at report that this was a mistake.

Placing, that is the spatial dimension of the ward, worked a sign system to be read and understood. In this way, naming and the spatial arrangement of patients, like the overall organisation of the hospital, acted to instruct and to enable the reproduction of the orders of the setting. However, nurses' identities and the identities of patients were also constructed through placing. Patients with no 'specific' nursing requirements were given to junior nurses and nursing auxiliaries to look after, while patients who needed high-dependency care and observation were given to more senior nurses to look after. The implication of these placements was that some patients' care *counted* more than others', was more important and difficult and required special skills and techniques. For the nurses, these patients had more status, as did the nurses who looked after them.

Sister: I do tend to leave the geriatric long-term patients to really middle grade nurses with an auxiliary ... second years, or occasionally first years, depending on the quality of students we have.
JL: Why and how do you make that sort of decision? What do you base that on?
Sister: Well, I tend to think that even most of the junior nurses know what basic nursing care is. They tend to know how to wash people, feed people, dress and just sit and listen to the older ladies. And I suspect they

would probably be a bit more frightened to look after somebody who's got central lines and IVs [intravenous infusions], although they do get an opportunity to do that as well, with the staff nurse.

Sister is justifying her practice of allocation and, through this account, reproduces particular identities and values which were present in the setting – junior nurses can carry out basic nursing care (washing, feeding, dressing and talking with *older* patients), but may feel frightened by the technology associated with and the expertise needed to care for the more sick patients. These relationships establish hierarchies of identity and values. Listening and personal care get down-graded to semi-skilled or non-technical work, while work with sicker patients is altogether of a higher quality.

This set of differences and identities relates back to the ward handovers, where what was observable and reportable were those aspects of patients which signified their medical condition or problems with mobilisation. Immovable patients were constituted as 'heavy' and were not particularly to be talked about. They were cared for but not looked after, where looking after is associated with the expertise of the extended medical gaze.

The placement of patients within the bays carried with it a complex of signals to be read in concert with other signifying and legitimating practices. These practices were configured around two aspects of nurses' discursive practices – notions of sickness and dependency, and notions of observation and surveillance. In the following section, ward routine and the materials which nurses use in their work are discussed and their role in producing ward life is considered.

Time, materials and routines: signalling care

'Ward routine', as described here, represents the carefully constructed events which help nurses accomplish and maintain the proper order of things. Routines not only get facilities to patients, but help organise the setting and the people in it in many more complex ways. The things that get included in routines are the 'taken for granted', almost invisible aspects of nursing work, the 'basic patient care'. But it is because routine care is unremarkable that it becomes useful in the work of differentiating and hierarchising patients, work and nurses.

Ward routine (the routine at the Royal University Hospital is described in Appendix 5) consisted of meals, nursing handovers, drug rounds, washing rounds, ward rounds, staff breaks, observation rounds, cleaning rounds, toileting rounds and bed-making. Not only did these events and encounters take place at particular times, but within themselves they were made routine; they were routinised[3]. It is within these routines that patients received particular forms of care – nurses sat a patient up in a chair rather than give them their meal in bed, helped them eat rather than leave them to eat themselves, gave them food from the trolley rather than a diet. The arrangements to ensure these differences were attended to were complex.

Nurses relied on their knowledge of patients from previous shifts and communicated these matters to each other as they paired up to do routine rounds. This was probably one of the single most crucial aspects of how nurses knew what to do for patients. The off-duty works so that on any one shift some nurses 'knew' the patients and nurses worked together to help each other know what to do, to pass on what they knew. This was not necessarily by verbal communication, but could be carried out through an action or a way of approaching a patient. When in doubt about aspects of nursing care nurses occasionally referred to the Kardex but, as already discussed, care plans were not used consistently, and instructions about care were not necessarily detailed explicitly. During the study it was noticed that the daily record would sometimes indicate whether a patient had been sat up the day before and this may have acted as a guide. The key is the 'status' or 'type' of patient, indicated via the handover where possible but also through the placing of patients in bays (see above).

Basic observations of vital signs were routinised. Most patients started off on four-hourly observations, decreasing to once a day over time as their condition settled. The night staff nurse ordered the observations. There was an observations book and any patient who needed more than once-a-day observations was written in this book. Some patients were on even more regular observations but this was specified for that patient and a separate observation chart was placed at the end of the bed, on the bedtable or on the locker. This gave it visibility. This extra observation helped signify that the patient was special in some way. According to the qualified nurses questioned in the study, the way in which the night nurse decided which patients should have what type of observation was influenced by the patients' condition, whether or not the observations had previously been abnormal (or for how long they had been normal) and the length of time they had been under observation. These aspects were not necessarily made explicit in the nursing records or at nursing handovers. These arrangements meant that the nurse taking the observations did not necessarily have any explicit explanation for why their patient was on these particular observations. They had to work it out by reading the signs and making connections.

Materials such as charts and equipment also help signify to nurses the things that need to be done for patients. For example, on their way round the ward a more senior student nurse or a staff nurse on the drug round may notice that a patient is on special observations. In the study, acutely ill patients were usually placed in bays 2 or 3. The records at the end of the bed (showing fluid balance, intravenous infusions, suctioning, nasogastric feeds, etc.) acted to tell nurses when the last nursing was done and sometimes when the next activity was due. Thus, equipment and charts acted to indicate or remind that care may be required once a nurse learned how to read the signs. The bays where more ill patients were placed were usually staffed by more senior nurses and they had learned to look out for these signs – they did not wait to be told.

The combination of materials and routines helps signal which activities will occur and how they will happen. For example, the arrival of a trolley announces to the ward the provision of a facility. Trolleys are used in the organisation of meals, drugs, drinks, linen, library books, tidiness, electro-cardiographs, doctors' rounds, washes, pressure area care and things to buy. Even death is announced to the ward by a trolley and the drawing of screens. Trolleys help staff to organise their work because they are sign equipment which work together with other signs, such as time. For example, I frequently saw a nurse bring a trolley with a bowl of water to a patient before any conversation about a wash had happened. This signals to the patient that they should sit up and get out their wash things. The arrival of wash trolleys, linen and wash bowls in combination with the time (after breakfast) all help signal that it is time for washes to commence. In these ways material artefacts help to signal care, and teach nurses and patients how to read the setting.

The day was marked out in time by routines. In this way patients automatically get care and nurses automatically know what to do once they know the routines, and the way to carry them through. In the ward studied, this was taken for granted. According to some of the qualified nurses, getting through the routines took priority above everything except emergencies. The individual, one nurse particularly felt, was sacrificed to ward routine.

The important issue is what aspects of 'care' or 'work' were routinised and what this told patients and nurses about the setting. Many activities in ward life were routinised and they occurred as repetitive activity, including patient admissions and aspects of the daily delivery of care. But rather than dismiss this routinisation as simply poor practice, routines emerged as critical to the ordering of ward life.

Paying attention to how nurses used routines helps further illuminate the hierarchies at play in the setting.

Nursing records

A detailed account of how the nurses in the study wrote their records can be found in Appendix 4. To summarise what is contained there, in their records the nurses made particular things about themselves and patients present, and others absent. Their records were their 'frontstage' accounts which kept in play what had visibility, while those aspects of work which were problematic were marginalised and remained hidden.

In the patient profiles nurses represented patients in relation to specified categories, such as hygiene, mobility, chest pain, temperature or self-care. The patient was thus fragmented into traits and parts. In the nursing records a patient's feelings and perceptions were rarely, if ever, recorded, except in relation to his or her physical response or as evidence of his or her 'behaviour'. Patients' wishes were rarely if ever mentioned so, overall, the patient was not figured by the records as an experiencing subject or as a competent agent. Rather, the patient was written in the nursing records as someone to be observed, as the object and subject of a nursing gaze. The records revealed that the nurses were bifocal. On the one hand they observed patients in relation to their medical condition, as the traces of disease to be deciphered by medical discourse. On the other hand, they observed patients in relation to their mobility and capacity to self-care. Both kinds of observation were noted in terms of a patient's progress and were used to signify their movement from illness back to health.

A patient was thus constituted as both a medical object and as the subject of a process – this subject should 'change' over time. The records showed that nurses were constantly alert to progress, or a lack of it. Therefore, in the way that they recorded, the nurses performed an extended medical gaze, a gaze concerned not just with the body of the patient as diseased but also with the patient's ability to function.

The records also said something about the nurses' own identities. For example, in writing their records the nurses did not use the first person, there is no 'I'. Although records were signed, the nurses constituted themselves as detached and objective rather than engaged with patients. In this sense, they 'figured' themselves as the 'eye' of the nursing gaze, but not as the sentient and experiencing 'I' of the cognitive subject, who sees, judges and decides, as represented by theoretical representations of nursing. The nurses' records thus circulated features important to the maintenance of both the clinical domain, and the need for patient mobility. Nurses diminished and effaced themselves and the patients as experiencing and competent beings and, in turn, diminished their own and the patients' authority.

The invisibility of caring at the bedside

Evidence of social relations between patients and nurses was absent from the records and handovers. As has been seen, more junior or unqualified nurses were not encouraged to pass on their understandings of patients derived from their close work with patients at the bedside. In the 'front-stage' spaces, at handover and in the records, nurses did not admit to treating the space at the bedside as a social space in which they enhanced their understandings of patients. These aspects of their work at the bedside were not made explicit.

Yet there were moments when these relationships were clearly of great importance. Nurses' conduct of care at the bedside conveyed more than the clinical world of calculation and observation created in notes and at the nurses' station. But these moments remained invisible and seemed to be entirely private. Such moments were constituted in the most mundane of nurses' encounters and often involved junior nurses or nursing auxiliaries. They also typically involved nurses doing something intimate with patients, such as washing, or simply in an acknowledgement of how the patient was as a person. Some patients, made vulnerable and laid low by illness, rely on the tact of the nurses in some of these most intimate moments. How these moments are handled are memorable and patients are grateful.

For example, in the following extract Mrs Adamson was behind the screens and had just stood up from the commode. It was the day after her admission:

> [Student nurse goes back in to the screens and Mrs Adamson is standing by the commode]
> **Mrs Adamson:** I'm sorry, I forgot to pull my pants down [she is trying to take them off and is panicky]. I'm sorry.
> **Student nurse:** Don't worry [soothing tone and helping Mrs Adamson to sit on bed and remove her pants]. I'll give them a wee wash for you.
> **Mrs Adamson:** I'm sorry, they'll be soiled.
> **Student nurse:** That's all right, these things happen to all of us.
> **Mrs Adamson:** I'm blooming useless.
> **Student nurse:** Don't worry.

In this extract the nurse helps restore Mrs Adamson's face with 'These things happen to all of us'. Her tone is soothing and her words help the patient to feel better about herself: 'I'm blooming useless', 'Don't worry'. In this way the nurse helps to cover the mishap and manage what Rudge (1997) has called a silence around the socially unacceptable disgrace of the body breaking its boundaries. This aspect of nurses' work also resonates well with Lawler's (1991) observations about the relationship between the hidden work of nurses in relation to those aspects of bodily existence which must also be hidden.

In the next extract Mrs Adamson had been having a breathless attack and was put back to bed, very agitated. The ward had been disturbed by another patient who had been screaming and attacking the nurses. This patient was admitted some days before, and had been very disturbed since that time. The nursing auxiliary comes over to Mrs Adamson's bed to tidy up:

[As she re-hangs Mrs Adamson's curtain the nursing auxiliary is speaking to the patient next to Mrs Adamson about the confused patient and how 'terrible it is'. She then steps down off the bed.]
Mrs Adamson: I'm sorry [conciliatory tone].
Nursing auxiliary: Ach! You didn't think I meant you, pet! Of all people! [she hugs Mrs Adamson]. Are you needing sitting up a bit? [A student nurse comes over and helps the nursing auxiliary sit Mrs Adamson up in bed].

In this extract Mrs Adamson's expression – 'I'm sorry' – indicates to the nursing auxiliary that Mrs Adamson thinks that she is the patient who is terrible. The nursing auxiliary exclaims and emphasises how could Mrs Adamson 'of all people' make such a mistake. The nursing auxiliary hugs Mrs Adamson and then, as if to confirm that Mrs Adamson is ill and an 'appropriate' patient, she notices that Mrs Adamson needs sitting up and helps to sit her up. In this small act of nursing care the nursing auxiliary reaffirms Mrs Adamson as a sick woman who needs care, and as some 'one' to whom she attends. She also reproduces the order of things – she is marking a difference between what constitutes the proper patient (really sick) and the improper patient (the demented and disruptive patient). In doing this she reaffirms her own identity as a nurse caring for the acutely sick and Mrs Adamson's identity as properly ill and worthy of care.

These moments do not lie outside the ordering of things. Inclusion is not as full persons, with authority. For example, within these moments the patient may be being confirmed as appropriate but as a medical object, not as an authority who can participate in processes of signification or legitimation.

The following extract is about Mrs Appleton. Mrs Appleton had been confined to bed having had a blackout which the nurses and doctors could not explain. Cot-sides were put on her bed and she was being observed. A student nurse had just been allocated to care for her during the morning. Although it was not mentioned at the handover, Mrs Appleton told the night staff that she was very anxious and nervous at being in hospital.

[Mrs Appleton is in bed, next to the nurses' station and she is trying to sit up without much success. She looks over to the nurses as they are getting up as they finish the nursing handover and catches the eye of the student nurse who is caring for her that morning. The student nurse goes over to the side of the bed and smiles. She bends down to the patient a little.]

Student nurse: Just try and lie back and relax [takes hand and smiles at Mrs Appleton. They talk for a moment]. Don't worry about anything.

Mrs Appleton: I get awfully upset.

Student nurse: We'll give you a wee wash later. Just try and relax and we'll get you back on your feet again. [Mrs Appleton visibly relaxes and smiles at the nurse, who smiles and goes.]

[Mrs Appleton lies back and closes her eyes. She is very fidgety still. The student nurse comes to the end of the bed with the back trolley. She pulls the screens round and takes the trolley in.]

Student nurse: There now you can have a good wash and feel better. You lie there – put your legs down – and I'll do all the work.

Mrs Appleton: I'm sore down there.

Student nurse: Are you sore down below?

Mrs Appleton: Uh-huh.

Student nurse: So what time did you come in last night?

Mrs Appleton: About six, and then up here about nine o'clock.

Student nurse: Give me your arm [she says this kindly in soft but confident tones]. Do you live at home by yourself?

Mrs Appleton: No, I live with my daughter.

Student nurse: With your daughter.

The student nurse reassures Mrs Appleton, not through telling her 'not to worry' but through letting her know that she recognises that Mrs Appleton gets awfully worried and that at this moment this is understandable. The nurse does not do the bedbath because she has been told to. At the handover she has only been told that Mrs Appleton is to have a wash and that she is to remain on bed rest. Frequently, in this situation patients are given a bowl to wash themselves with minimal help, but the nurse is translating the instructions into something more than a 'wash in bed'. She is doing a full bedbath. Giving patients a bedbath, with full back trolley, is a sign – it tells the patient or an onlooker that the patient is so ill that they cannot or must not do anything for themselves. The nurse 'takes over'. She does not ask why Mrs Appleton is trying to get up or has caught her eye but tells her 'to lie back and relax'. She is confirming Mrs Appleton as ill.

When the patient tells the nurse she is 'sore down below', the nurse does not pursue this as a lead but goes on to ask the patient about who she lives with. The nurse does not enter into a conversation about the soreness down below and in this way Mrs Appleton is denied participation in the authoring of her troubles. It is only Mrs Appleton's clinical identity which is confirmed as someone who is 'very ill' and 'very worried'.

Mrs Appleton and Mrs Adamson were confirmed as appropriate to the current setting, as *really* sick. The disorders of their bodies and their ineptitude were exonerated. They were confirmed in the notion that it was the illness, and not them, that led to these displays of diminished responsibility. Such moments between nurses and patients are confirmatory but only because, in them, nurses and patients join together to reaffirm the proper order of things. These occasions do not escape, they are still socially organising. In addition, such moments of care at the bedside also indicate all the work that nurses do not make visible, all that they know about their patients which never gets talked about. The nurses knew that Mrs Adamson and Mrs Appleton were frightened and anxious, that they were sentient beings who needed care and what used to be called TLC.

Discussion

This chapter has shown how ward life is ordered and disciplined through some of the nurses' routine activities, including their discursive practices. The division of labour, nursing records, nursing handovers and the placing of patients act in concert to relay that certain aspects of patients have more importance and can be talked about as significant, while others are less important and remain unspoken. In other words, the way in which each feature of ward life is managed has an expressive and performative dimension through which the orders and meanings of the setting are circulated. These can be understood as power effects.

The handovers, nursing records, ward routines and the temporo-spatial organisation of ward life help to produce and circulate systems of signification and legitimation, identity and difference. Through these practices 'accountability' is constructed. Following Garfinkel (1967) accountability refers here to what is observable and reportable. In this way the facets of nurses' practices discussed in this chapter circulate what forms of activity are legitimate (for example making medical sense through observation of a patient's behaviour) and the aspects of patients that are significant (for example their blood pressure rather than their experiences).

In this way of circulating significance records and handovers relay to nurses how they are to conduct themselves. For example, nurses learn from the handovers how to attend to the patient as an object constructed by the extended medical gaze. They also learn that they sometimes need permission, from doctors, protocols or less clear sources of authority, and that only certain sources of authority have permission to speak (or write) certain things. Critically, the patient as an experiencing subject, by their very absence from the handovers and records, emerges with little authority. While care at the bedside acknowledges the patient as a sentient being, it denies either the patient or the nurse the authority to decide what is significant.

Nurses emerge as the *conductors of care*. But, like orchestral conductors, they are not free to decide how ward life should be ordered or care conducted. Like electrical conductors, nurses are the conduits through which power effects are made possible. In privileging acutely ill patients who require observation and technical care, nurses keep themselves visible as skilled and knowledgeable. But they are also complicit in the effacement of their other less visible work at the bedside when they care for patients as sentient beings.

Nurses' organisation of the clinical domain depends upon a continuous labour of division. Patients and junior nurses have no authority. The authority to speak comes with the discipline of the medical gaze. This ongoing labour of division is present in every aspect of nurses' work, from the placing of patients to the use of routines. Through it, nurses differentiate patients, types of work and types of nurses in relation to hierarchies of significance. Thus, to fabricate the clinical domain, nurses engage in 'a constituting of classes'.

The next chapter focuses on nurses' relations with doctors to examine how this constituting of classes facilitates the production of the clinical domain as well as the managerial objective of a flow of beds.

Notes

1. A 24-hour tape is a recording of a patient's heart activity over a 24-hour period which helps to diagnose the relationship between abnormalities of the heart rhythm and exertion. A small electrocardiograph is attached to the patient. During the investigation the patient is supposed to behave as normally as possible.
2. Erect and supine blood pressure: nurses take a person's blood pressure while they are lying in bed, then get them up, standing or sitting, and take another reading of blood pressure. In some conditions the body cannot maintain its flow of blood to the brain and the blood pressure drops considerably, causing the person to be dizzy or faint. This is called 'postural hypotension' and it is associated with a variety of pathological conditions, as well as old age.
3. For Giddens (1984, 1991) routines represent regularised and repetitive action – a continuity which is essential, not just in terms of the reproduction of institutions, but also to personal identity. At an existential level Giddens argues that routines give a feeling that what is happening is 'under control'; this helps impart a sense of ontological security. Routines also represent an economy of effort (Berger & Luckmann, 1966). Berger & Luckmann suggest that through

making particular practices unreflexive and habitual, attention and creative capacity are freed up to enable concentration on aspects which cannot be attended to through routines. I want to stress a different aspect to routines: nurses allocate some aspects of care to routines, and in doing this they differentiate the mundane and everyday aspects of care from the more important and technical or expert aspects of care which are made to appear extraneous to the routines. Further, in the nurses' handovers, deviation from routines requires justification (Berg, 1992). But only some grounds can be drawn on to support an account or a deviation, such as doctor's orders.

Chapter 4

The Nursing–Medical Relationship: Moving Patients through the Medical Domain

Introduction

As the previous chapters have illustrated, nurses are the conductors of care. Yet they are not free to decide what care should be given, or how. Nor is it the case, as is sometimes asserted, that nurses simply follow orders. Yes, nurses regulate themselves to align with managerial concerns for increased throughput, and they work with doctors to accomplish first class medicine, but not because they are forced to do so. It is all much more complex than that.

These observations raise the question as to how medicine is distributed between nurses and doctors. And what does this distribution accomplish in terms of the ordering of the medical domain? As indicated in Chapter 2, it is argued that the ward round is a 'spectacle' which exemplifies and recreates an appearance of first class medicine. Like the front entrance of Royal University Hospital, the ward round celebrates and reaffirms the reputation of medicine. It maintains the appearance that the operations of medicine are purely technical and disciplined matters which are held apart from the social. Through the ward round the particular character of first class medicine is made present and dominant in the lives of nurses and patients.

Nurses appeared to attend the ward round in order to inform doctors about their clinical observation of patients and to keep abreast of how the doctors viewed the patients. But the ward round was also concerned with keeping patients moving through the medical domain. This work involved much more than visualising patients as medical objects; it depended upon nurses' work of contextualising patients' troubles. However, nurses' contributions were made to disappear from view on the ward round and so the round located the nurses to the 'back stage'[1].

The chapter begins by describing doctor–nurse relationships[2]. It goes on to examine consultant ward rounds and the social round. Nurses' work of contextualising patient troubles and monitoring their progress provide some of the grounds for moving patients through the medical domain. Even though nurses' work contributes to the flow of beds, the way in which ward rounds are conducted causes that work to be effaced.

Consultant ward rounds

Doctors' ward rounds were attended by the senior nurse on duty who was the nurse in charge at the time of the round. Each consultant did a ward round at least once a week. If the consultant was 'waiting' (that is, responsible for admissions) then he or she would do a ward round on the admissions ward and on their 'own' unit the day after 'waiting day'. Some consultants would also do another ward round the next day if this was over the weekend. A lecturer, senior lecturer, registrar or senior registrar attended the patients with the resident doctors most days. This ward round was not scheduled and a nurse did not always attend it.

Consultant ward rounds were spectacular occasions. Typically, they were organised as follows: the consultant and their team (residents, attached medical students, lecturers, senior lecturers, medical registrar and any visiting doctors) congregated somewhere on the ward and then went round each patient under their care. Sometimes the consultant talked to or examined the patient at the bedside, and sometimes he initiated discussion about the patient at the notes trolley at some distance from the patient. Importantly, the ward round remained public and visible throughout, except when a patient was being examined, when the screens are drawn around their bed.

For 'new admissions', the resident read out his 'history' and the results of his examination of the patient to the consultant, indicating any investigations already or about to be undertaken, and giving any results obtained. This was done either at the bedside in the presence of, but not including, the patient, or at the notes trolley, standing in the middle of the ward or at the end of a bed.

The consultant then sometimes examined the patient and talked with the patient. The consultant then discussed the patient with the other doctors and they decided on the diagnosis and future 'management' (tests, investigations, treatment or discharge issues). In respect of elderly patients, the doctors were alert to viewing patients in relation to their 'functional' and social situation (how the patient usually managed at home and any possible longer term difficulties, such as urinary incontinence) and these matters sometimes entered their discussions at the ward round.

Asymmetries in power relations

On consultant ward rounds studied at the Royal University Hospital, nurses rarely participated in discussion about patients. Like patients, they acted passively. Nurses positioned themselves discreetly, taking notes and occasionally responding to questions about their observations of patients or offering perfunctory agreement to plans made during the doctors' discussions. The nurse accompanying the ward round typically stood on the periphery of the group and very rarely spoke unless she was asked something specific by one of the doctors. Typically, she did not initiate any discussion nor did she volunteer information.

The following extract was taken from a 'waiting day' ward round. The extent of the questioning is unusual but illustrates the aspects of nursing work which nurses are asked to report during a ward round.

[Mrs Appleton, day 2. The ward round is congregated at the end of Mrs Appleton's bed and Mrs Appleton is lying in bed. She has had two episodes of collapse this morning. The staff nurse is on the ward round.]

Consultant [to staff nurse]: How is she now, dear?
Staff nurse: She's much better.
Consultant: How often has it [the blackouts] happened?
Staff nurse: Twice.
Consultant: What time was that?
Staff nurse: Between 8 and 9.
Consultant: And in between she's been quite all right?
Staff nurse: She's been feeling faint and tired.

The consultant is addressing the staff nurse as a witness: she is giving evidence and is questioned to help establish the facts. He uses closed questions to elicit information. This specifies the focus of the staff nurse's responses and delimits her participation to matters as directed by the consultant. This example also illustrates how nurses act to extend the medical gaze. Their surveillance of patients is an aspect of their work which is legitimated by the medical. Through it not only do patients become visible, but their own activities have visibility as being purposeful because they are in support of the medical process of diagnosis and treatment. The extract also indicates the nature of nurses' participation in the ward round – it does not represent a discussion between two different occupational groups with different views of the patient, but between occupational groups where one of which (nursing) works to support the other (medicine), and which appears to have a similar viewing lens as medicine. Further, it should be noted that the nurse's behaviour in relation to the patient at these times did not support any notion that she was there as the patient's advocate or partner.

So far, it would seem that the relationship between doctors and nurses is asymmetrical. Some nurses spoken to during the study were certainly dissatisfied with their relationship with doctors, but they said that this was because they were not always kept fully informed, rather than that they saw things differently from doctors. These are very troubling issues. But rather than leave it that nurses are subservient and passive underlings, I want to push the research material further and ask a different question: what do the ward rounds accomplish?

First class medicine: Mrs Marsh

The two areas of nursing work which nurses were asked to report on at ward rounds were their observations and their work to get patients moving. As noted in Chapter 3, these are the same aspects of nurses' work which were talked about in detail at ward handovers and reported on in their written documents. Therefore, one aspect of nurses' *visible* work on ward rounds was to contribute to differential diagnosis and attest to a patient's progress and recovery as the (implicit) outcomes of medical intervention and nursing care.

But examination of ward round procedures makes it clear that decisions about diagnosis and discharge were taken along with the wider contextualisation of a patient's troubles provided by nurses. In these ways the ward is a key site for accomplishing (and circulating) the two agendas of a continuous and adequate flow of beds, and the appearance of first class medicine. The following extract illustrates this.

[Mrs Marsh, day 3. Mrs Marsh is sitting by her bed in a chair in bay 2. She is wearing her night-dress, dressing gown and slippers. The ward round comes into bay 2. Present are the consultant, lecturer, senior house officer, two residents, two research fellows, two medical students and Sister. They stand by the notes trolley in bay 2.]

Resident [to consultant]: Mrs Marsh [indicates patient] – the pea lady.
Consultant: Is she new?
Resident: She came in the day before yesterday [he reads from the notes and looks up at the consultant as he speaks. He speaks quietly, confidentially and the others stand around]. Essentially, she swallowed a pea at lunch time and became increasingly wheezy by the evening. By 8 o'clock she was very breathless and so phoned her GP who sent her in here. She settled with nebulisers [a method for moisturising and prolonging inhalation of a decongestant]. She's been having daily

physio. Her drug history – she's on warfarin [a blood thinner] because she's had a number of DVTs [deep vein thrombosis] in the past, but no pulmonary emboli [clots in the circulation to the lungs]. She's on tamoxifen [mild, oral chemotherapy for breast cancer] for a lump in her breast but I can't find it.

Consultant: Have you got the old notes to see what goes on there?

Resident: No.

Consultant [looks at lecturer]: Let's get hold of the old notes and check up on what's happening here [turns back to resident].

Resident: There's some old myocardial ischaemia [damage from constricted blood supply to the heart] with some failure. She's fine, she lives alone. On systems enquiry she has some ankle swelling. She is apyrexial and she has had a . . .

Consultant [interrupts]: So there is nothing of serious note on inquiry?

Resident: No.

Here is a 'properly conducted' medical exchange. The resident presents the evidence in a quiet and confidential manner and the consultant checks that all that should be done is being done. As a managerial device the ward round can constitute a form of inspection and audit of both doctors' work and aspects of nurses' work. This is first class medicine in progress.

But on looking again there is more going on. The resident calls Mrs Marsh the 'pea lady', a strange, metonymic device. Doctors and nurses frequently call patients by their medical parts ('the appendectomy', 'the MI', 'the bunion'). But Mrs Marsh does not get identified in this way, which would at least figure her as 'medical'. The resident says she *swallowed* a pea and then became breathless, hours later, thus requiring a doctor. An ambiguity is brought into play here. Swallowing is the *normal* thing that should be done with a pea and no breathlessness should result. He then says that since she came to hospital she has had very limited treatment. The machines tell the doctors that Mrs Marsh has a little old heart damage, and a little bit of heart failure, and the consultant sums up with there being 'nothing of serious note'.

So Mrs Marsh's identity is in the process of being transformed – she is being moved from being someone who is potentially acutely ill to someone whose underlying problems are chronic and mild. And further, she is being discredited as a witness because she claimed, according to the medical notes, to have *inhaled* a pea.

[The consultant then walks over to examine the patient himself. He gives her a big smile.]

Consultant: Hello Mrs Marsh, I am Dr Fox [he shakes Mrs Marsh's hand].

Mrs Marsh: Hello.

Consultant: How are you feeling?

Mrs Marsh: Well this hurts like mad – they gave me an injection [she shows him her arm all bruised]. It is terribly painful, I don't want any more of those.

Consultant [looks at others who stand around]: What is that for?

Resident: Bloods.

Consultant [laughs, he's crouched down by her now]: Well, hopefully we won't have to do any more of that now.

Mrs Marsh: Now I'll ask you the question everyone asks you – when can I get home?

Consultant: We'll see about that. Now, have you been coughing at all?

Mrs Marsh: No, wheezing.

Consultant: How long have you been wheezy?

Mrs Marsh: Just the once when it happened.

Consultant: And are you still wheezy?

Mrs Marsh: Yes, not as much except with the machine. That makes me wheezy.

Consultant: Have you been coughing up any spit at all?

Mrs Marsh: No.

Consultant: And when you walk around do you get short of breath at all? [He is looking into her eyes and listens intently to her replies.]

Mrs Marsh: I don't walk far – no not really.

Consultant: And at night – how many pillows do you use?

Mrs Marsh: One around here.

Consultant: Can you lie flat?

Mrs Marsh: No, but I don't have a lot of pillows.

Consultant: Do you stack them up?

Mrs Marsh: No.

Consultant: Do your feet swell up at all? [He looks at her feet and legs.]

Mrs Marsh: I have had that for a long time.

Consultant: I've seen your X-rays and they are all right but they are not completely normal – there is a bit of infection there. Now we're wondering whether to do some more tests or not. Do you live alone?

Mrs Marsh: Yes.

Consultant: And do you manage on your own?

Mrs Marsh: No. I have a home help three times a week and friends and family help me.

Consultant: I see, I'll go and look at your notes and have a think what to do [he pats her hand and smiles].

The evidence is amassed and displayed and the patient is made visible. The consultant's physical examination is not extensive. This particular absence marks how he is not figuring Mrs Marsh as very ill – a very sick patient is confirmed as very sick through the extent of the consultant's physical examination of them. Mrs Marsh, however, may not know this. Rather, she would see how thoroughly he checks the evidence produced by others, the resident and herself included, thus emphasising his role as the 'expert', as embodied authority. He proceeds in a closed question and answer format, giving very little feedback to the patient as to why he's asking these question or what the significance of these matters is. He thus ensures that he controls the turn-taking. This process does not only include the medical evidence of any pathology, or the possibilities of pathology, but also the patient's 'social situation' – 'is she safe at home, 'how does she manage?'. This aspect of this phase in the process is important, because the patient's chest X-ray is not normal and they may want to do some tests. They could do it on an outpatient basis but there is a slight risk involved if she is not supported well in the community.

Mrs Marsh, however, is far from being the passive participant one might think. Indeed, she is particularly plucky. She complains about her arm being painful and states she will not have any more injections. She also questions the consultant on her own initiative with 'Now I'll ask you the question everyone asks you – when can I get home?'. However, the consultant politely but firmly puts Mrs Marsh in her place. He laughs and, with the authoritative and (if you are one of his colleagues) inclusive 'we', reminds her who is conducting the discussion ('we' hopefully will not have to do any more injections and 'we' will see about when you can get home).

The effects of the consultant's questioning can not be explained simply as an example of the maintenance of medical dominance. By persistently focusing on Mrs Marsh's ankles, how many pillows she uses at night and how far she can walk, the consultant, even in the face of the ambiguity raised by Mrs Marsh's responses (such as that she only uses one pillow at night which would normally indicate an absence of heart failure), indicates that Mrs Marsh's signs and symptoms may be due to chronic problems, exacerbated by the current episode, perhaps, but nothing too serious. In this he follows the resident's lead and confirms the original picture: Mrs Marsh is the pea lady, with nothing serious of note.

In the next phase, when the consultant moves back to the notes trolley, by 'thinking out loud' he gives a stunning performance of due medical process, in which all the relevant facts are weighed up and considered.

[The consultant goes back to the notes trolley and moves up the ward, well away from Mrs Marsh. The others follow.]
Consultant [to lecturer]: What are we going to do? I don't want to take her off the tamoxifen. Presumably she is on it for a good reason. We

need to get her notes and check up on that. And it seems a pity to bronchoscope her. She is in mild heart failure?

Lecturer: She's had frusemide [a diuretic].

Consultant: How much?

Resident: 40.

Consultant: Well, we'll increase that.

Resident: [nods]

Consultant: My feeling would be to let her go home and then bring her back in 10 days to outpatients where either you or Dick could see her. She could have another chest X-ray then. And you could decide if she needs a bronchoscopy [use of a tube to visualise the insides of the lungs].

Lecturer: She's got no temperature.

Consultant: She's asymptomatic. She may have a touch of LVF [left ventricular failure] with this nocturnal dyspnoea [shortness of breath] business. We could send her home on diuretics and you can see her in outpatients in 10 days time. If it's not all right then you can broncho-scope her. I should think a cooked pea would disintegrate – I should think it would be disintegrating and might just leave a shell. [To Sister] I'll let her out, it sounds as if she would be happy to go home.

Sister: Oh fine – yes.

Consultant: We'll send her home on 80 of frusemide then? [To resident] And is she on antibiotics?

Resident: No.

Consultant [to lecturer]: And the diagnosis – what would you say? Dyspnoea of unknown cause with mild LVF?

Lecturer: [nods]

Consultant [to senior house officer]: Are you happy with that, Geoff?

Senior house officer: I haven't had anything to do with this lady.

Consultant: Oh, I'll just go and speak to her.

The consultant arrives at a decision: the pea should disintegrate and the patient can go home and be followed up in outpatients. He refigures Mrs Marsh as having no medical future and as having no disease effects which are amenable to medical intervention. Before finalising any decision he seeks consensus, but only *after* he has indicated the way forward. Each member of the team who counts is asked if they are happy with his reading of the situation and with his solution. If they are not happy they have to contradict him and indicate other possibilities in front of the others. So, while he gives the appearance of collaboration, he actually gives very little room for any other point of view. It would take a very trusting team for one of them to contradict him or argue for a different way of seeing Mrs Marsh (see Goffman, 1958, on trust and tact). To help tip the balance, he enrols Mrs Marsh's own desire for knowledge about when she can get home.

The last phase of the performance is to notify the patient that she can go home and to get her agreement.

Consultant [speaking to Mrs Marsh]: So we think you could get home – would you like to go today?

Mrs Marsh: Oh, not today. My family are at a convention and they won't be able to bring my clothes in until tomorrow. There is no way of contacting them.

Consultant [looks at Sister]: All right?

Sister: That's fine.

Consultant: Good, home tomorrow. We'll see you in outpatients and check the wheeziness has stopped. We'll give you some water tablets to take home with you. And you can go tomorrow, that'll give your family a chance to bring in some clothes for you. All right?

Mrs Marsh: Thank you very much doctor.

[The consultant smiles, pats her hand and leaves. As he walks off the lecturer speaks to him.]

Lecturer: What about the salbutamol?

Consultant: Well, if it hasn't helped much, stop that and give her a larger dose of diuretic and see her in outpatients. [To Sister] Are you happy with that Sister?

Sister: Yes, fine.

Mrs Marsh's transformation, a return from patient to person, and her disposal are almost accomplished: she can go home but not until the following day because her family are not available. But there is more than this: Mrs Marsh's medical disposal depends upon her troubles being reconfigured as inappropriate to the acute medical domain. This is accomplished by contextualising her troubles (wheeziness, etc.) so that the 'evidence' is moved around to suit a diagnosis which casts doubt on the authenticity of the patient's claims, that she choked on a pea. The revised diagnosis of dyspnoea with mild LVF is important in this context. Asthmatics with mild heart failure do not need to be in hospital but they do get wheezy, especially at night, and they have swollen ankles. Mrs Marsh is transformed from someone with an acute episode and potentially at risk to someone with chronic heart problems (due to old age) which she in fact denies.

The consultant only refers to Sister after his deliberations and once the patient's discharge is in sight. Even then, it is an indirect referral, more for confirmation of his reading of the situation than anything else. The consultant gives Sister the opportunity to add anything once they move away from the patient after the decisions have been made. So it appears that Sister is only deferred to once the important work of medical decision making has been accomplished. The consultant is, tacitly, relying on Sister – it is she and her nurses who are charged with the work of assessing Mrs Marsh in relation to her mobility and the resources she has at home to support her. Any doubts about her readiness for discharge could be raised here or would already have come to the doctors' attention through less formal channels. But Sister is also the only person on the ward round in a position to know the exact bedstate. She has the overview of when people are being discharged from all the consultants' teams. In this instance, it is the consultant's waiting day the following day and it is important to free up the beds.

Importantly, while the medical gaze seems to operate in a rational and reasonable manner, there is a subtle and present assumption in the consultant's conduct towards Sister, that Sister has assessed the patient in relation to her mobility and that if she was particularly worried by any aspect of this patient her assessment would have already informed the medical view. Significantly, it was possible to trace in the research material that Sister had indeed already come to the conclusion that this patient was ready for discharge *before* the ward round[4].

Later, on the day of the ward round, the shortage of beds became explicit, and Mrs Marsh was sent to another ward for the night and discharged from there the following day. She made her own discharge arrangements, including contacting her home help to restart.

The example of Mrs Marsh helps to illustrate how a new, more streamlined health service might be accomplished. It is not that Mrs Marsh did not have problems, it is just that her troubles were reconfigured as inappropriate to the acute medical domain. She was shifted from a category of patient whose troubles were appropriate to a category whose troubles were inappropriate to the medical domain. The point is just how ambiguous the matter of medical diagnosis is. But it is Sister who provides the context in which the consultant is willing to take the risk.

Mrs Adamson and the flowers: returning patient to person

Around Mrs Adamson's admission there was a small possibility of difference between the nurses' view and the doctors' view. This was concerned with whether the patient had psychosomatic problems or was 'really ill'. Here is the first ward round concerning this patient:

[The ward round comes into the bay. Present are Sister, a consultant, two medical students, a resident and a senior house officer. The consultant goes straight to Mrs Adamson. He crouches down by the patient as she lies in bed and takes the patient's hand. He smiles.]

Consultant: Hello, Mrs Adamson, my name is Dr Brown. Just sit quiet while they tell me about you. [He looks up and the resident comes and crouches next to him and speaks very quietly. He reads from the notes and gives a very brief resumé of the patient's history and examination.]
Consultant [to Mrs Adamson]: Let me have a wee listen to your chest – just open that one button for me. [The patient undoes the button on her nightdress and the consultant puts on his stethoscope and listens to her chest. Sister pulls the screens round and the rest of the ward round stand at the end of the bed.]
Consultant [stops listening and turns to look at the senior house officer]: I can't hear much in the way of crackles. [Turns back to patient] Well love, I think we'll do three things for you [he's taken her hand again]. First – you just relax – you're in the best place possible. Second, we'll give you a wee bit of oxygen – would you be more comfortable with a nasal tube rather than the mask? Does it make you claustrophobic? [Mrs Adamson doesn't really answer.] We have a kind of nasal spectacle – have you ever had nasal spectacles?
Mrs Adamson: I wear spectacles but I haven't got them with me.
Consultant: No, these are a different kind of spectacle. It's a tube that puts the oxygen up your nose. We'll give you some medicine to help you get better. You rest quiet and look at the beautiful flowers in the sunshine [he points to the flowers on the windowsill – a lot of them are dead or dying].
Mrs Adamson: Yes, it's a lovely day.
Consultant [he gets up to go and pats the patient's hand. He speaks to Sister]: Can we give a bit of that now [pointing to the oxygen mask]?
Sister: Yes, of course.
[The consultant walks off and Sister puts the mask on Mrs Adamson. The ward round moves off and the senior house officer speaks to the consultant as they walk back to the notes trolley.]
Senior house officer: She's had attacks of breathlessness in the past – they couldn't find a cause and put them down to anxiety.

Sister makes two contributions to the round: she draws screens around the bed to enable privacy while the consultant examines the patient's chest and she signals that she has received the consultant's direct instructions to give the patient oxygen immediately. But there is more being communicated than this.

The consultant's conduct puts the patient in a passive position: she is lying in bed, she is patted and smiled at but told to be quiet, she is not asked anything except if she has had nasal spectacles before, and she is told that three things are going to be done for her to make her better (one of these she is to do herself – relax.) Meanwhile she is to lie quiet, and 'look at the beautiful flowers in the sunshine'. The consultant, through his talk to the patient, indicates his view of the situation and implies how this patient is to be managed. In raising her need to relax and her potential claustrophobia, he draws attention to Mrs Adamson's anxiety. At the same time he confirms that she is ill and that she needs to be looked after carefully – she needs to be kept quiet and relaxed, she needs medicine and oxygen, now. His manner is demonstrably caring and concerned (albeit paternalistic).

Through his emphasis, the consultant puts into play two possible grounds for the explanation of Mrs Adamson's troubles: one is somatic, and appropriate to the place, an acute medical ward, and the other is psychosomatic and chronic and is not suitable to an acute medical ward. The GP's letter provides the basis for Mrs Adamson's troubles to be explained on other than purely medical grounds. The letter stated that Mrs Adamson was well known to the practice. She suffers from chronic anxiety and frequently calls the surgery. The letter indicates that this patient's symptoms, breathlessness and chest pain, are usually due to her anxiety. She is being figured as neurotic and as always bothering the GP. But the letter also indicates that the current episode is different – the GP states 'she is clearly unwell at present'. On her arrival in A&E she is described in the admission document as 'very distressed' and 'cyanosed', with lungs full of fluid. Her chest X-ray and ECG confirm that she has heart failure and a probable heart attack. At this point then the machines and the doctors are Mrs Adamson's allies: they help to keep interpretation of the effects she displays in the acute medical arena, but only just.

Sister stands back as a virtual non-participant on the ward round, as is usual. She is not consulted and her view of the patient is not sought, nor is it offered. Sister has to decode the consultant's behaviour and can take or leave what she has been told. The process relies on her attention, her ability to decode and her self-discipline. The significant aspect here is that the consultant does not directly discuss this patient's mental or emotional state with Sister, and that she does not raise it. There is no record of the ward round in the nursing notes and Sister does not hand over to the next shift. Nothing is made explicit at first as to how Mrs Adamson is to be handled.

Throughout Mrs Adamson's stay the nurses kept in play the ambiguity over the cause of her troubles. At first, the nurses were very kind to her when she was distressed and having an attack of breathlessness and chest pain. But their ambivalence to her became more overt as Mrs Adamson's medical condition seemed to stabilise. The stability of Mrs Adamson's condition was constructed by the nurses' readings of Mrs Adamson's body, which returned to normal even though Mrs Adamson's troubles remain unresolved. The shift in the nurses' talk to a more overt scepticism was exemplified by the staff nurse's handover to a late shift:

Staff nurse: Mrs May Adamson, 85-year-old Church of Scotland lady who came in on the 22nd with an MI, complicated by left ventricular failure and atrial fibrillation [an arrhythmia of the heart]. She's having apex and radial pulse done [where the pulse is taken at the wrist and the number of heart beats are listened to and counted at the same time to see if they synchronise]. They think it's just a complication of the MI. She's just had stat. doses of digoxin [digitalis, to calm and slow the heart rhythm] – she's not having it regularly. She's on frusemide [a diuretic] regularly. She has pulmonary oedema [fluid in the lungs]. She has odd turns. There's no doubt she has chest pain but we're not sure if it's as bad as she says. She looks fine one minute – like just now, she's really perky – then she's terribly breathless and [mimics someone gasping for breath]. She can have GTN [glyceryl trinitrate to dilate the coronary blood vessels in angina pain] for chest pain. She needs a lot of reassurance, you know. She had to have Cyclimorph [a preparation of morphine and an anti-emetic] this morning – five milligrams IV. David Trent [the lecturer] said we're not to hesitate to give her Cyclimorph if she needs it as it's good for her LVF [heart failure], apparently. I don't know how it works. This is her third day. She's just been up to sit before lunch, for lunch in fact. But she had one of these episodes of breathlessness and chest tightness this morning so she just got up to sit before lunch. Her weight is coming down, which is good. And her apex and radial are synchronising this morning.

The staff nurse aligns a heterogeneous array of matters to make sense of Mrs Adamson's persistent troubles. She aligns Mrs Adamson's age, the doctors' conduct towards her, the fact that she is permitted Cyclimorph, the patient's own erratic conduct and the machines' objective gaze (the apex and radial pulse and the patient's weight.) The staff nurse relays how the patient is getting better. This progress is indicated by Mrs Adamson's weight reduction (a sign that her pulmonary oedema should be resolving), and the synchronisation of her apex and radial heart beat (a sign that her heart arrhythmia is settling). But the staff nurse cannot balance these observations with the 'episodes of breathlessness and chest tightness'. The staff nurse is not sure if she can believe that physical illness alone has caused the effects Mrs Adamson displays. She makes the doubt explicit: is the patient's pain as bad as she says it is and is her visual distress from breathlessness 'real'? She uses the doctors' conduct to help her interpretation: David Trent (the lecturer) has said Mrs Adamson can have Cyclimorph if she needs it – a sign that she is legitimately ill. But something does not quite add up for the staff nurse and she cannot quite believe the patient's distress (her 'odd turns') but she has to because 'illness' is being legitimated by the medical staff's approach and care. However, through her different explanations she communicates her doubt.

During the study, the tests and other objective measures of Mrs Adamson's body functions began to return to normal and her attacks were reclassified as psychosomatic and, as such, something the patient could help rather than being caused by illness. The nurses' conversation about her changes – she no longer has chest pain and breathlessness, but is said to 'hyperventilate', and have 'palpitations' and 'panic attacks' – describe the psychosomatic affects of anxiety, not the effects of somatic heart problems which would be 'breathlessness', 'arrhythmias' and 'distress'. There was also a marked change in the nurses' behaviour toward Mrs Adamson.

While Mrs Adamson was figured as 'ill', the nurses spent a lot of time reassuring and comforting her. But as she was refigured as having psychosomatic problems, the nurses seemed to question the time which reassuring her and nursing her took. Here, for example, is Sister helping the patient out of bed six days after her admission:

[Mrs Adamson is behind the screens doing her morning wash. Sister goes in and asks her if she has finished and pulls back the screens. She's in a big hurry.]
Mrs Adamson: Before you pull back the screens dear I think I'll need the . . .
Sister: Loo? [pulls curtains back round].
Mrs Adamson: I'm sorry.
Sister: That's all right [she goes and fetches commode. They're both behind the screens].
Mrs Adamson: I'm sorry, dear.
Sister: Take nice deep breaths, none of these silly little pants. [Sister's voice has a hard edge to it, authoritarian or irritated.] No! Slowly, slow down – right [her voice begins to soften]. That's better, good [her voice is soft now]. What's wrong?
Mrs Adamson: That water tablet.
[The nursing auxiliary goes in behind the screens and she and Sister come out together and leave. The screen is left half pulled round. Sister returns and goes into the patient, helps her off the commode and into her chair and pulls back the screens. Mrs Adamson is sitting in her chair with her head in her hands, puffing. Sister opens the windows on the other side of the patient's bed and leaves.]

In this episode Sister is short and indicates she has no time to spend on Mrs Adamson's 'panic attacks'. She says 'take nice deep breaths, none of these silly little pants' and she opens a window.

By this time any 'ordinary' heart attack patient would be mobile and independent if not actually discharged. In this exchange, Mrs Adamson was returned to person, a deeply anxious person, who panics and gets breathless.

Shortly after this episode, Sister and the doctors on a ward round decided to send Mrs Adamson for convalescent care. She was discharged there three days after this extract. She returned to the ward a few days later, having continued to have her attacks at the convalescent home. The nurses kept her mobile. The day after her readmission she had a cardiac arrest in the bathroom and died on the floor.

Throughout her stay Mrs Adamson was figured as someone who needed reassurance and her anxiety state was always held in view. As the objective tests returned her body to normal, and time ticked by, the nurses were able to reattribute her breathlessness and chest pain to the effects of anxiety, not as its cause. The nurses kept in play their indecision over the ground upon which Mrs Adamson's troubles could be interpreted and, by doing this, it was possible for them to shift the ground upon which her troubles could be explained. Thus, they were able to transform her identity. This shift was important as it allowed Mrs Adamson to be reconfigured as someone for whom the nurses were not fully responsible because she had chronic psychosomatic problems, not acute medical problems. However, I am not suggesting for a moment that this is a heartless or uncaring process.

Mrs Adamson had problems which did not go away. The nurses drew on her social and medical history to shift her identity and get her moving. It was through their attention to the non-medical aspects that the nurses were able to contextualise this patient's troubles. Therefore, it seems that it is nurses who continuously balance a patient's needs with those of the service to continue the flow of beds.

Pulling patients through the beds: surveying the social

Nurses contextualise patients' troubles and monitor their progress through the beds. This work is intimately connected with nurses' work of pulling patients through the medical domain. At the hospital in the study, the nurses' interest in the movement of patients through the beds was most explicit in the social round, the round conducted by the geriatrician in Sister's office. In this, the *social* domain, Sister seemed to have a much greater say than she did in the clinical domain of the ward round. To illustrate this, in the following extract, Mrs Best is being discussed at the social round for the first time since her admission. The consultant geriatrician saw her and had done an 'assessment' of her at the beginning of the week (this was also a part of his own research program).

[Attending the meeting are the consultant geriatrician and his senior registrar, two Sisters, two physiotherapists, two occupational therapists, two residents, a speech therapist and a social worker.]
Consultant geriatrician: Ann Best?
Senior registrar: She's still here.
Resident: Her barium shows she's got a large benign ulcer. She's been put on Gaviscon.
Consultant geriatrician: Is it a gastric ulcer?
Resident: I haven't seen the films yet and they didn't say over the phone.
Consultant geriatrician: From the social point of view, she lives with her daughter and gets out and about with her.
Sister: Yes, I think she'll just go home.

The consultant geriatrician leads the discussion of this patient with a question and the resident updates him on the medical situation. The consultant geriatrician checks if it is a gastric ulcer but the resident cannot qualify at this stage. The consultant geriatrician then sums up what he has assessed about this patient in terms of the 'social point of view': she 'lives with her daughter and gets out and about with her'. Sister agrees with this, and concludes the discussion with 'she'll just go home'. So here it is Sister who concludes the projected discharge on the basis of her albeit unspoken assessment.

The smooth discussion is full of signals: this patient has a medical condition for which there is no radical treatment (she is 80, the ulcer is benign, surgery is out of the question), and she has a daughter who looks after her in the community. On the ward she is termed 'self-caring', is figured by the nurses as mobile and is able to wash and dress herself. From their assessment of this patient there is consensus: no further intervention is required and there should be no impediment to her discharge.

The purpose of the social round is to discuss fully each of the older patients in relation to their medical diagnosis and treatments, their rehabilitation and their social situation, but only in respect of how any of these may impede their discharge. For example, the presence or absence of relatives living at home or the frequency of visits by home help and other community workers act as signs which can be read to indicate how fragile the older person is at home. Where there is a high frequency of home visits staff infer that community support is already stretched to breaking point, without the added weight of any new illness and subsequent disability. These matters are not used to help focus on a patient's current needs. So the question remains, what are nurses and doctors assessing at these meetings, if it is not actually a patient's 'condition'?

It appears that they are contextualising a patient's troubles in ways which help them to assess a patient's potential for a medical future. This in turn depends upon how easily they can be discharged. The round brings to light impediments to a patient's discharge and helps ensure that all possible care is taken to mobilise resources to enable as speedy and safe a discharge as possible, in whatever form this might take. The rounds also help to keep in play other possible non-medical explanations for why a patient may not be getting better. To illustrate this, here is an extract from a social round in which Mr Gibbon is being discussed. Mr Gibbon has been assessed as having social problems because his wife is an invalid and his own health is poor. They have community services to almost maximum support. The nurses have informed the doctors that Mr Gibbon is proving difficult to mobilise. In this exchange, the doctors have been trying to decide why Mr Gibbon is slow to get moving.

> **Senior registrar:** I got the impression things are pretty hefty at home, with his wife and all.
> **Resident:** She's in and out – she's psychotic I think.
> **Senior registrar:** She goes to the day hospital, doesn't she?
> **Resident:** Yes, but there is some psychiatric history.
> **Senior registrar:** She may be demented?
> **Resident:** No, she's a very dependent personality, that's it. Also she's a cancer phobic.
> **Senior registrar:** Right, okay, he's really a medical problem. The home help five days a week is more for his wife than for him.

At the same time as the geriatrician keeps in play the social as a possible ground for explaining Mr Gibbon's sluggishness, he holds Mr Gibbon on the medical ground: 'he's really a medical problem'.

This move was critical as it sent the ward doctors back to review Mr Gibbon's diagnosis. A few days later the senior house officer reinterpreted a routine chest X-ray to rediagnose Mr Gibbon – he had had pneumonia for some time and there was some suspicion that he had cancer. This accounted for why he was so tired. The doctors were no longer concerned to find out about his mood because they now had an explanation for his sluggishness and they told Mr Gibbon that they would send him home as soon as possible so that he could go on looking after his wife. The patient began to recover when he was moved to the side ward, started on antibiotics, and given something to help him sleep.

Mr Gibbon's social problems were disposed of. The doctors did not medicalise his home life and the geriatrician did not allow ward staff to socialise his medical troubles. The nurses were satisfied as the patient was on the move. Critically, by holding the interpretation of Mr Gibbon's troubles on the medical ground, the limits of the clinical domain were also redrawn – they were not social workers but acute care practitioners.

The social round exemplifies the new form of examination and history through which a patient's home life, their 'social situation', as well as their behaviour gets surveyed for signs. Nurses emerge as central to this process. But, critically, the social round also helps hold the processes of clinical medicine apart from the social, to maintain the appearance that clinical decisions are taken on purely clinical grounds.

Pushing patients through

Medical decisions seemed to be taken with the nurses' contextualising work already informing doctors' views. The senior nurses begin calculating a patient's potential for movement from the moment of their arrival in the clinical domain. Here to illustrate the point is the case of Mrs Weston.

In the following extract, Sister has taken the handover from the staff nurse who accompanied the patient on her transfer from the admissions ward. Sister had no contact with Mrs Weston at the time of her arrival, but stands at the end of her bed to take the transfer. The transfer centres on the admission document and on the technical equipment attached to Mrs Weston to enable observation of her vital signs. These include a central venous line (CVP) and a urinary catheter attached to a urometer. Sister comes over to see Mrs Weston about 40 minutes later and looks at the urometer with the student nurse assigned to look after the patient. Mrs Weston is on hourly measurements of urine. Sister moves next to the patient to speak with her.

> **Sister** [moves over to patient and leans down]: How are you feeling? Is your shoulder sore?
> **Mrs Weston:** My leg.
> **Sister:** You got a bad knock yesterday – can you remember what happened?
> **Mrs Weston:** I was at the island and crossing the road when the car came and hit me ... [inaudible] ... I am usually so careful. I didn't see him.
> **Sister:** Ach, well, don't worry [she takes the patient's hand].
> [Mrs Weston goes on speaking as doctors arrive at the bed and Sister turns away. The patient continues to speak, turning to me.]
> **Mrs Weston:** ... a policeman came over on the other ward but I ... [Sister and the doctors walk off].

Sister asks how the patient is feeling but immediately qualifies her question to focus and limit the patient's response to whether or not her shoulder is sore. Sister may have been asking the patient what happened because she wants to check whether the patient is suffering from any loss of memory and to get an idea of her general state. In other words she may have been masking her intentions. At the arrival of the doctors, Sister turns from the patient who is in mid sentence. Her turning away from the patient as the patient is speaking indicates she is not particularly interested in Mrs Weston's own version of events. A little later Sister accompanies the lecturer on his examination of the patient. She spends quite some time on this and from this consultation she takes away 'information' about how Mrs Weston is to be 'managed' according to the doctor (the patient can drink and is to remain on hourly measurements of urine and central venous pressure). For the time being the medical staff are figuring Mrs Weston as acutely ill.

At the handover following the patient's admission, Sister reads from the records that the patient 'was knocked down yesterday by a car'. Sister reports that Mrs Weston 'is fine' and can be 'up to sit'. This seems to contradict how the lecturer is figuring Mrs Weston. A staff nurse then points out that 'they' are mobilising patients with the particular kind of fracture which Mrs Weston may have suffered (there remains some uncertainty of diagnosis here), and Sister's response is as follows: 'Yes get her going, get the physios to see her. She's 88 – we ought to get her going'.

In her assessment of the patient, that she is fine, and in her directive to 'get her going' Sister appears to be attending to some other, absent discourse which makes aspects of Mrs Weston's situation significant and which legitimates her directives. In doing this she over-rides the junior doctor. However, from the observation data Mrs Weston was far from fine. She exclaimed, moaned with pain and attempted to resist when the nurses, including Sister, wanted to move her so that the doctor could examine her chest. She quite clearly told the nurses and the doctor that any movement was 'very sore'. Further, Mrs Weston was evidently concerned and shocked by what had happened to her, as can be seen in the exchange with Sister about being hit by the car. However, Sister did not mention the patient's feelings about her accident and while she takes the 'pain' into account it is in an oblique, disembodied way. She did not describe the patient's pain but only discussed analgesia, in terms of her own assessment of the patient's pain:

> Sister: She's for all care, turns two-hourly. And for paracetamol. Analgesia ... she's written up for Cyclimorph but I think that's a bit fierce really – ask them to write her up for something less powerful, DF118 maybe. She's fine. She can be up to sit.

At the beginning of the handover Sister described the patient to the assembled nurses as 'a new patient, Mary Weston, 88, who I do not think is a medical problem at all but an orthopaedic one. She is an RTA [road traffic accident].' In doing so Sister reduced Mrs Weston to a metonym, 'an RTA', and to an organisational problem, 'an orthopaedic' one. She is to be mobilised, because she is '88'. Sister successfully refigured Mrs Weston, even in ways which contravened medical orders. Later, in conjunction with the geriatricians, Sister arranged for Mrs Weston to be transferred to a rehabilitation unit for older orthopaedic patients. In Sister's assessment, Mrs Weston constituted a threat to the flow through the beds and this was spotted early rather than late. Mrs Weston's clinical needs were subsumed under the need to refigure her as someone who should be mobilised, someone who needs to be got moving, early rather than late. To do this Sister refigured Mrs Weston as 'other' – Mrs Weston was inappropriate because she was not an acute medical patient but an orthopaedic one. It was not that Sister did not care, she just had organising work to do.

On another occasion Sister accompanied a senior lecturer to the bedside of an elderly lady who had been immobilised by chronic chest problems, coupled with pneumonia for over three weeks. The lecturer told Sister to have the patient walked to the toilet and he said 'kill or cure'. Sister arranged for her to be walked to the toilet. The patient died that night.

Discussion

The division of labour between doctors and nurses hides a distribution of medicine which is complex. Nurses and doctors work together to sustain the flow of beds and to achieve and demonstrate medical outcomes (i.e. progress and recovery). But the relationship between doctors' diagnoses and nurses' assessments of patients is far from one of succession.

While consultants' ward rounds are key occasions for accomplishing and circulating the orders of the clinical domain, nurses' conduct is not the direct effect of doctors' orders, nor are nurses dominated by doctors. Both doctors and nurses are engaged in configuring and, importantly, reconfiguring patients' identities. Their work together enables particular patients to access medical and nursing care. That is, both doctors and nurses work to distribute medicine as an important social resource. This said, the parameters and definition of what constitutes medicine are also constructed by the work that nurses and doctors do together. This is the second way in which nurses and doctors distribute medicine. Frontstage, doctors (with the exception of geriatricians) perform those aspects of patient assessment that make it appear that a medical decision is taken on a purely clinical basis. Backstage, the nurses' work of observing, exploring and interpreting a patient's 'social situation' provides the context, which in turn affects medical decisions.

Nurses *contexualise* patients' troubles. In some cases where there is the potential for a blockage to the flow of beds, they may also help maintain an undecidedness over the grounds upon which a patient's troubles can be interpreted. Maintaining this undecidedness over interpretation helps provide the *mobility* necessary to keep patients on the move. This is important in an environment where a patient can stay acutely ill only for so long, as in the case of Mrs Adamson. Thus, nurses' assessments affect diagnosis and diagnosis itself is a moveable feast that depends, to some extent, upon the wider context of a patient's troubles.

This effect has been exemplified in extracts concerning Mrs Marsh and Mrs Adamson – both of them had troubles which were 'refigured' as the consequences of biological decline or psychosomatic illness, rather than as the effects of acute illness. These sorts of moves provide the flexibility necessary to keep patients moving through the beds.

Yet the ward round and doctor–nurse relationships are instituted to efface the contextualising work provided by nurses. It is kept virtually invisible. Effacing nurses' contextualising work has three important effects. First, it helps maintain the appearance that diagnostic and discharge decisions have been taken on a purely clinical basis. The dirty work of socialising troubles is kept separate from the work of clinical decision making. Second, it maintains the supplementary, rather than complementary, status of nurses' work. Third, effacing nurses' work as 'non-clinical' renders it as 'other', and as 'social' rather than technical work. Thus, effacing this contextualising work does not just efface how medicine is distributed between doctors and nurses but is another instance of how the constituting of classes is maintained and circulated.

It seems then that it is nurses who are made to appear as the ones who press the organisational need for movement and flow, the dirty work of the clinical domain. It appears to be nurses who pull patients through the beds. In the cases of Mrs Adamson and Mrs Weston, the potential for disagreement signifies that it is nurses who carry the burden of getting patients moving. In the cases cited, the nurses got Mrs Adamson and Mrs Weston moving while the doctors faded into the background. However, both these patients were not very good medical materials. In reality nurses are helping to accomplish the medical agenda of having patients who are good for first class medicine, patients who can be seen to recover, patients who can be seen to be processed. Those patients who block the flow are also those patients who do not fit the medical bill. Because nurses' contribution to the dirty work of organising is visible, it is *their* identity which risks being downgraded. In taking the brunt of these polluting aspects of hospital work, nurses help maintain the purity of the clinical domain as the doctors' prerogative.

So how do nurses conduct their relations with patients, given these restraints? The next chapter addresses this issue and explores nurses' relationships with patients around the time of their arrival in the acute medical domain. While these relationships appear very institutionalised, on closer analysis nurses' conduct helps initiate patients into the clinical domain so that they know how to conduct themselves to maintain their inclusion as appropriate clinical materials.

Notes

1. The distribution of medicine between doctors and nurses mirrors feminist discourse which points to the ways in which the interdependence of the public and the private domains is kept invisible (see also Davies, 1995).
2. There have been many theses concerning doctor–nurse relationships, including the notion that there is a doctor–nurse game (Mackay 1989), in which nurses pretend that they are not influencing doctors' decision making in order for them to be able to do just that. More often than not the doctor–nurse relationship is figured as one of domination. Historical studies by Davies (1995) and Rafferty (1996) suggest that nurses are rendered intellectually and materially subordinate to doctors because of the gendering of knowledge, work and organisation through which nurses' work and knowledge are feminine and thereby culturally downgraded. The current study overlaps with these analyses, but suggests that it is not doctors that nurses are subordinate to. Rather, doctors and nurses (as well as the rest of us, see Lupton, 1995) are 'subordinate' to the discipline because its associations with positive knowledge make it a strong ground, readily available for circulation and performance. The difficulty is the matter of ownership: doctors hold responsibility for some decisions and the distribution of resources, and perform medical decision making in ways which make it appear as if they alone make the decisions. This chapter disturbs that assumption.
3. The consultant ward round was usually the only occasion upon which senior nurses and consultants meet to discuss patients. And even though the middle grade doctors had coffee in Sister's room with some of the qualified nurses, they rarely if ever, in my presence, conversed about patients or their work together. More typically doctors talked to each other, about football or other concerns, and the nurses sat perched on the arms of chairs and observed this display of the doctors' social life. There would also be some low-key flirting and sexual innuendo. Where just junior doctors had coffee with nurses there was more conversation between them.
4. At the nursing handover on the day the patient was admitted, Sister reported the patient's extensive medical history and her age. At this news, the staff nurse at the handover heaved a great sigh of discontent, but Sister turned to her and told her that the patient was 'not bad'. The following morning at the nursing handover, Sister expressed the view that the patient could end up with a lung abscess if the pea was not extracted. But after a morning in which she had a chance to observe Mrs Marsh, Sister stated at the midday handover that the

patient 'should be ready to go home soon'. Mrs Marsh during this morning shift had been able and had shown herself to be willing to be mobile and to be self-caring.

5. Mrs Adamson, throughout her stay, made cracks about being for the mortuary and told me that she was terrified of what the pain and palpitations might really mean. While in hospital she had two complications from her heart attack – heart failure and atrial fibrillation – both of which would exacerbate any tendency to breathlessness and palpitation. Why Mrs Adamson reacted so badly to them is a question that was not raised; she was a known neurotic any was old, the concern was whether or not they were authentic, not what her experience of them meant to her. She told me that normally she could not manage stairs without getting a breathless attack, and that because of them she had not been going out for two years. She claimed that any exertion threw her into a state of breathlessness or brought on the pain in her chest.

6. In summary the ward rounds can be described as having several dimensions. First, they are functional – they are about reviewing and accumulating evidence to enable prompt diagnosis and decisions about treatment to keep things moving, to facilitate diagnosis and treatment issues. Berg (1992) has termed these 'medical disposals'. As the Professor of Geriatric Medicine put it in an informal interview with me, the ward round served as a time 'for evaluation', 'to keep exit always in mind', 'to stop things drifting'. The ward round at this level constitutes a form of inspection and audit, of both doctors' work and aspects of nurses' work.

Second, they are ceremonial. As a ceremony, the ward round is confirmative (Turner, 1967) to help produce and reproduce the power relations of the hospital. Through the conduct of the ward rounds (the placing of the patient and the different members, the routinisation of turn-taking) and through dis-cursive practice, identities are confirmed. Importantly, the social is held apart from the medical as a purely clinical domain and the division of labour and the distribution of medicine between nurses and doctors is accomplished.

Third, the ward round is a ritual through which transformation (Turner, 1967) of a person into a patient of a particular type and, critically, their return from patient to person to enable their discharge can be accomplished. This entails an ascription of patients to classes: patients are ascribed to a class, which acts as permission or instruction to deal with patients in particular ways. These classes configure around constituting a patient's 'troubles' as either somatic (acute or chronic), social (age is also constituted as an aspect of the social), or psychosomatic.

Classifying patients helps facilitate their disposal. Disposal can be literal, in the sense of accomplishing shifts in a patient's identity so that they can be discharged, as in the case of Mrs Marsh. Or disposal can be metaphorical, in the sense that staff dispose of their responsibility for patients because they are rendered or figured as inappropriate to the acute medical domain. There are some patients, such as Mrs Adamson and Jessie discussed in Chapter 2, whose problems might be so serious and long-term that they are simply not going to go away. The nurses can only dispose of patients literally by disposing of them as the objects of their concern and responsibility. By reconfiguring their clinical identities, nurses shift them into categories of patient (the chronically sick, the psychosomatically ill) for whom they do not consider themselves responsible. In this way nurses help accomplish a patient's literal disposal and the disposal of the nurses' own feelings of responsibility towards them.

Chapter 5

Nurses' Conduct: Initiating Patients into the Social Organisation of the Medical Domain

Introduction

This chapter explores how nurses conduct their relationships with patients. The focus is on the period at and immediately after a patient's arrival to the ward. Nurses refer to this period as 'admission'.

Importantly, the admission procedure, the filling in of forms, is not in itself constituted by nurses as their assessment. But, as we will see, the admission procedure fills an important role – nurses' conduct of the admission period initiates patients into the social organisation of the medical domain.

Through their encounters with nurses, patients learn how to conduct themselves to maintain their inclusion as clinical materials. Critically, patients must efface themselves as social beings to be rendered appropriate medical objects. This includes allowing others to authorise their needs. Patients learn that 'authority', to define what is significant and to legitimate action (Giddens, 1984), lies far from the bedside and not in the nurse–patient relationship.

The first part of the chapter describes how nurses operationalise the admission procedure. The second part of the chapter presents a nurse–patient admission interview, to demonstrate how nurses' conduct helps initiate patients into the world of first class medicine.

Doing admissions

The admission period is the time allotted to the deliberate or procedural collection and documentation of information about a patient. Nurses refer to their activity around a patient during this time as 'doing an admission' or 'admitting a patient' (not as assessment or diagnosis). A nurse is asked to 'admit' a patient and new nurses are shown how to 'do an admission'. Nurses construct the admission around the completion of the patient profile or 'nursing record' (Appendix 4). Typically, they do not carry out any nursing care during this period.

How the ward nurses complete the formal admission process varies according to where the patient has been transferred from, how ill the patient is and his/her apparent ability to communicate. The main points of the admission process are the completion of a patient profile, including baseline observations such as temperature, pulse and blood pressure, checking any property through the property book and putting it away in the locker allocated or arranging with a relative for its removal, filling in and applying a wristlet nameband, and filling in a namecard and placing it above the patient's bed. The admission is also 'put through the admissions book'. This is the ward record of all patients who are admitted to the ward with some basic details, such as name, address, age and diagnosis.

If a patient is admitted via another ward the nurses do not do a full admission. Instead they do baseline observations, check and record property but omit the interview with the patient. Nursing records are transferred with patients from other wards, and even where this nursing record is incomplete, the nurses do not go through this part of the procedure with the patient. In the study it was noted that for patients transferred from the admission ward the profile was hardly completed at all.

Typically, one nurse is given responsibility for admitting a patient. Sometimes she is helped by another nurse with a specific aspect of the admission, such as taking a patient's observations or putting away a patient's belongings. The nurse admits on the basis of the geographical location of the patient on the ward. Student nurses are very rarely helped directly by the qualified nurses unless it is their first admission.

Nurses allocated to admit patients use several sources of information to fill in the profile. They consult the admission document, referred to as the 'pink slip', and typically transfer information such as the reason for admission, medical history, past medical history and provisional diagnosis directly onto the nursing records. Nurses do not usually consult any previous hospital notes, which are taken to the doctors' room, off the main ward area, at or shortly after a patient's arrival. The resident doctor takes a patient history after the nurses have done their admission of the patient so that the doctor's 'in-patient' clinical notes are also not available at the time the nurses admit the patient.

When a patient has been transferred directly from A&E, the admitting nurse does a type of interview with the patient. Occasionally, a nurse interviews a patient's family or relatives as well as, or instead of, the patient. Relatives are interviewed by nurses away from the patient's bedside, usually outside in the corridor leading to the main ward area where they are left on the patient's arrival to the ward. This occurred in the case of four of the elderly patients in the study. It transpired that this was done because the nurses perceived each of these patients as possibly 'confused'.

The 'interviews' with patients take place with the patient in bed and the nurse either sitting on the bed with the forms on her lap, standing at the bedside with the forms on the locker, or sitting in a chair at the bedside. Admitting nurses do not introduce themselves by name to the patient prior to the interview. The admitting nurse usually checks the patient's demographic details, fills in the details on the profile and fills in the wristlet nameband and places this on the patient's wrist. Thus, the patient is labelled. The nurses never make a formal, systematic physical examination of the patient at the time of admission but do take 'baseline observations' (the patient's temperature, pulse and blood pressure). The nurses do not weigh or measure the height of patients on admission.

Thus, the very ways in which the admission period is typified and structured indicate that it is a procedural, institutionalised event, rather than an important occasion for discovery and interpretation. The admission of patients is now discussed in greater detail, first in terms of how admissions are organised by nurses and then in relation to how interviews with patients and their families are conducted.

Effacing the social

'Admitting a patient' commences prior to a patient's arrival on the ward. In A&E the patient is undressed, their clothes and their other belongings put in a large plastic bag and, usually, a hospital gown is put on them. Paperwork has already accumulated and is transferred with the patient to the ward. Paperwork consists of an admission document, any old medical notes from previous admissions, and any letter from their own GP.

Where family accompany a patient, they are told to wait outside the ward on the patient's arrival (this is also an aspect of the procedural rules as defined in the manual, see Appendix 6, point 8). Thereafter, the family's access to the patient is restricted by nurses and by the rules of the hospital. Visiting times are usually restricted to an hour in the afternoon and an hour and a half in the evening. Exceptions and privileges are sometimes granted by nursing staff. For example, the family of patients who have just been admitted might be allowed access for a time after the patient has been examined by the doctors. Here, for example, is an extract from Mrs Menzies' admission:

[The visitors' bell rings]
Student nurse: That's for the end of visiting time.
Mrs Menzies: Oh, is it?
Student nurse: Yes, visiting time is between three and four in the afternoons. Is that your daughter outside?
Mrs Menzies: Yes.
Student nurse: I'll let her come in when we've finished – she can stay on. You're privileged today [smiles].

The admitting nurse tells Mrs Menzies that she is 'privileged' because her daughter can come in to see her, the nurse will 'let' her in. The nurse is indicating how special permission is required for family to have access to patients outside the prescribed times. For patients who are no longer being 'treated' by medical staff, the dying and the long-term, family might be allowed to visit at any time, but this, of course, relies upon these patients being constructed as 'dying' or 'long-term' in the first place. Such matters are not, as has been discussed in earlier chapters, self-evident.

Much of the sign equipment that people use in their presentation of themselves in their day-to-day lives is removed on their arrival. Clothes and jewellery are designated 'property', listed and put away or taken away by family. Even a patient's family is restricted from access. In this sense, patients are denuded, sometimes literally, as in the case of Mrs Violet, whose pants were left down. Critically then, control over a patient's access to belongings and family is transferred to nurses during the admission period.

Patients' autonomy is eroded through the strict procedural and bureaucratic structure of the admission. Typically, patients are not asked during the admission period if there is anything they want to keep with them, if there is anything or anybody they think they might want or need before their things or their family are packed away or sent off. These decisions are made on their behalf by the nurses. To counteract them would require work or protest by patients or their families. For example, here is an extract from Mrs Appleton's admission. It is just after eight o'clock in the evening. Mrs Appleton, having arrived about ten minutes before, is in bed being interviewed by the student nurse.

Student nurse: Did anybody come in with you?
Mrs Appleton: Yes, my daughter – she's waiting outside.
Student nurse: Will she take your clothes home for you?
Mrs Appleton: Yes.
Daughter [comes in at this point and stands just inside curtains, picks up plastic bag of property]: I'll just pop home with these, shall I, and bring in your night things?

Mrs Appleton: Oh, yes.
Student nurse: Oh, you don't need to come back – are you coming in tomorrow?
Daughter: Yes, in the afternoon.
Student nurse: Well, it'll wait until then. We can lend her a nightie for the moment and we've got little packs with soap and things in.
Daughter: Oh all right then. I'll just go now, shall I? You don't need me, to know anything?
Student nurse: No, we're all right [smiles].
Mrs Appleton: Yes, don't trouble yourself. Behave yourself [smiles].
Daughter: Right [hesitates at curtain]. Bye.
[The student nurse is writing on forms and the daughter leaves.]

Mrs Appleton and her daughter live together. It can be seen in this extract that the student nurse takes over from Mrs Appleton and her daughter in deciding what Mrs Appleton needs: she can wait until tomorrow to have her things brought in and they do not need the daughter. The student nurse has only just met Mrs Appleton and may have little idea of the sort of things she may need or of the kind of person she is – whether, for example, Mrs Appleton wears spectacles or would appreciate her daughter coming back as a comfort at a stressful time. The daughter hesitates, and checks if the student nurse needs her to know anything, but the student nurse says 'no, we' will be all right. This exclusion of the daughter may have been an attempt to include the patient. If 'we' denotes herself and the patient, then the student nurse is now constituting them as aligned in some way. But, at this point, she has a limited relationship with Mrs Appleton because they have only just met. Further, the 'we' is ambiguous, it may also be an institutional 'we' – we, the doctors and nurses, do not need you to tell us anything that we need to know.

Mrs Appleton's daughter telephoned the ward from home some time later to let the nurses know that her mother gets 'agitated'. A nurse came over to Mrs Appleton at about 10 pm to tell her about the call. The night nurse told Mrs Appleton that her daughter has said that she gets agitated, but did not attempt to discuss this with her and she did not stop to listen to Mrs Appleton telling her about how she feels. The nurse disposed of the problem by reassuring the patient that she is 'safe' and that the nurses are 'close'. She presumed a relationship of trust, and that the patient would feel better if she was made to feel safe, by knowing that the nurses are close. But, like the student nurse, this nurse and the patient have only just met. By behaving in this way the nurse avoided engaging with Mrs Appleton through not allowing Mrs Appleton the space to express herself.

According to the night nurses, Mrs Appleton became very distressed in the early part of the night. The night nurse explained that Mrs Appleton's behaviour was possibly due to the fact that she sometimes takes a sleeping pill and may have had 'withdrawal'. Her vulnerability from agitation was not passed on as an aspect of her 'profile' to be treated as a part of her nursing care.

Other patients, like Mrs Appleton, appeared disconcerted by a loss of control at these times. For example, Mrs Gardner and Mrs Violet both questioned the location of their property and they appeared not to trust the people involved to look after their things for them and ensure their safe delivery. In the case of Mrs Violet, her daughter returned with a bag of things for her while she was being examined by the resident doctor, but the nurses did not let her know and let the daughter go home without seeing her mother. Mrs Violet expressed disappointment at this. Where family could be useful in providing information they were 'included' for a time and questioned by staff. This usually happened in the cases where there was some doubt about the patient's state of mind.

This exclusion of family and control over their access to patients was a systematic and regular feature of how the nurses dealt with family. It was one of the ways in which nurses detached a person from their social selves to transform them into a patient. While these processes are, in one view, disempowering for patients through the nurses' conduct of care at these times, patients learnt that if they were to get on in the setting they had to permit their transformation from person into clinical object.

Structuring admissions

Nurses' conduct announces that patients are now in the hands of those around them and that, for the time being, the person as a social self is subordinate to the needs of the body as constructed and defined by medical and nursing discourse. There are many different aspects of nurses' conduct which, in concert, accomplish this movement in a patient's status. A few aspects are discussed below to serve as an illustration, but this is not an exhaustive account.

First, although patients are the centre of activity they are positioned through the activities of others. This process was illustrated by Mr Dean's admission. The receiving nurse, the porter and the transferring nurse took the decision about how to get the patient into the bed, they did not ask the patient. These strategies helped position the patient to be *displaced* as socially potent. In this way patients are not figured as participants who have the authority to say what it is that they want or need.

Second, acute admissions are routinely put to bed. Putting the patient to bed and immobilising them at the beginning of their stay enables access by doctors for their examination and 24 hours of bed rest gives the doctors a chance to see how the disease takes its course in the body as a 'treatment space'. There is a parallel discourse available which indicates that prolonged immobility is bad for the body, especially for older patients. So patients are also routinely got up after 24 hours, or sooner if they are older. These arrangements are not usually discussed with patients, they are imposed. As we have seen in Chapter 5, patients are expected to comply with these arrangements. Where patients do not or cannot comply, they are figured as unable to conform to the orders of the medical domain; they cannot efface themselves as a social being.

Third, nurses rarely introduce patients to the place or to those present and they rarely introduce themselves, by name or by rank. Not knowing who people are puts the patient at a further disadvantage, leaving the patient to work it out for themselves. This is because knowing what institutional roles people occupy gives some indication of their power to help you so not knowing who they are can help to exclude. For example, Major Stevenson, a retired major and accustomed, as he told me, to 'being in charge', was aware of this. He stressed the need to know people's names. At the end of his admission interview he asked the admitting nurse and myself our names and, later on in his stay, he asked me to tell him who all the different people were and what their uniforms signified, because 'I have no idea to whom I'm speaking – whether it is someone with the power to help me, the authority, or not'.

Fourth, nurses' conduct sweeps patients along in the flow of the nurses' agenda. As already stated, patients are typically not asked what *they* need or want. During the admission period the nurses seem to postpone attention to patients' immediate requirements unless these are legitimated by authorities coming from beyond their relationship with the patients. Adherence to procedural aspects at the time of the admission appears to take priority over response to immediate issues arising out of the patient's condition (for example resting, thirsty, needing a wash, needing to go to the lavatory or having something to eat). Typically, nurses attend to issues which can be established as 'needs' through drawing on an available discourse. Nurses do not prioritise any immediate requirements that emerge during the admission period through their proximity to or their conversations with patients. For example, in the case of two patients transferred from the admissions ward the morning following their admission, the patients were sat up in a chair shortly after their arrival. In both cases the patients had been admitted during the previous night, were in their eighties and had, by their own account, hardly slept at all. However, the nurses gave the patients no real choice in the matter and got them up to sit in a chair.

Nurses' conduct relays to patients that they have no authority to legitimate their own needs or nurses' activities, and that they must concede to other authorities, far from the bedside. The very way in which nurses complete the patient profile and take their history of the patient helps define these as the orders of the setting.

Form-alities: method and the constitution of meanings

The nurses structured their admission of patients around completion of the nursing profile and this included an interview-type encounter with patients and/or their relatives. The purpose of the admission procedure was to enable a 'history' of the patient to be constructed.

The wording of the procedure manual (Appendix 6) implicitly directs nurses to the type of approach they are to take – they are told that 'any *information required is obtained* from relatives' and to '*collect* and document *necessary information*'. The wording is revealing. It supports the notion that the admitting nurse, the patient and their family do not participate in the constitution of what is 'required' or 'necessary', but are sources from which information can be obtained or are the instruments through whose agency data can be collected. It is important to point out that the admission interview is not being constituted as an interactive and interpretative event, through which nurses, the patient and their family arrive at an understanding of a patient's needs and how these are to be addressed. On the contrary, the patient is being rendered a discrete object about which certain things need to be known.

This framing of the admission interview was reflected in the way in which the nurses announced it to patients. Only on one occasion was a nurse seen to introduce herself and it was her first admission. Nurses sometimes gave no explanation of what they were going to do and just started to ask the patient questions, but with the forms prominently to hand which they filled in as they went along, and which may have announced that their questions were part of some bureaucratic and legitimated procedure. Sometimes nurses did give patients an explanation of what they were going to do. On one occasion a patient was told by the nurse that she was going to 'check some details', in two instances patients were told that the nurses were going to 'admit' them, and on another occasion that the nurse was going to 'ask some questions'.

In these ways nurses announced to patients that filling in the form is what is on their agenda. They did not give any indication that they were uncovering details that might affect the way they were going to nurse the patient. The interview was constructed as a procedure to be completed with the patient's assistance, not a conversational arena in which the nurse and the patient could talk about the patient's health or their current experience to ascertain what nursing was required.

The nurses conducted the interview very much as if the patient profile was a structured questionnaire. They usually led the interview and turn-taking was set at a question and answer format. During the admission interview the nurses did not seek patients' narratives and they typically refused anecdotal forms. This method of interviewing can be considered a 'discursive genre' (Fairclough 1992), which constitutes both the inter-viewer and interviewee in particular ways. The interview is constituted as an aspect of a process carried out on the patient, not as an exploration or as a form of discovery to be undertaken *between* patients and nurses. But there is a further significance. As we have already seen, the procedure manual instructs the nurse to obtain from patients and their relatives 'information' as 'necessary' or 'required'. These terms are not completely ambiguous but support the underlying epistemology of the setting, that within the setting there will be specific types of information that it is necessary to know, but that the status of the information is not arrived at in conjunction with the patient. There are facts which need to be revealed and only then can interpretation take place. Patients and relatives are constituted as helping reveal the facts but not as involved in their inter-pretation. Interpretative expertise is located outside the nurse–patient relationship; that is, the centre of discretion lies elsewhere.

Sticking to facts and defining need

The interview was structured like a questionnaire and followed the sequence given on the profile. Nurses controlled the direction and the areas covered in interview. In their questioning of the patient, nurses avoided speculative investigation of a patient's experience and under-standings and they got patients to 'stick to the facts'.

Aspects of the patients' way of living were medicalised. For example, patients were not asked about their appetite, how they took their meals, how they cooked, what kinds of food or drink they consumed or how their weight has been. Rather, they were typically asked if they were on any 'special diet'.

Similarly, patients were asked what medication they were taking. Nurses are responsible for giving the patients their medication so knowing what medication a patient is taking might have acted as a cross-check on the doctor's prescription (such as if he had included all the patient's usual drugs and at the same doses and, if not, why not). It may also have been a check on what was wrong with the patient. But nurses did not ask the patient how taking the medication affected them.

Nurses also focused the interview on 'problems'. They announced to the patient that they only wanted to know if the patient had a problem that had something to do with the condition that they were in hospital for. They were in effect asking the patient to make their own assessment of matters. This was done through the use of leading questions. For example, patients were asked if they had a problem with their bladder or their bowel:

> **Student nurse:** Do you have any bladder problems?
> **Mrs Violet:** Only during the night. As I said, I get up every two hours, but during the day I'm all right.
> **Student nurse:** Any bowel problems?
> **Mrs Violet:** No, I'm a good girl. I take All Bran every day for breakfast.

Here, the student nurse restricts Mrs Violet's replies to any problems the patient may have. Although Mrs Violet gives the nurse details about how her bladder disturbs her during the night and how she takes All Bran for her bowels (implying some potential difficulties), the nurse does not explore these issues further. Sometimes patients were told ahead that they did not have a problem:

> **Staff nurse:** You get out and about, you're fully mobile, you don't need a stick or anything?
> **Mrs Mitchell:** Oh, no.

The staff nurse gives the patient no chance to tell the nurse about how she 'moves' about: staff nurse has made an assessment and tells the patient that she does not have a problem with getting around. She makes several moves – in the first, she translates the dimension of 'getting around and about' into a medicalised version ('being fully mobile'). She then uses metonymy to reduce the issue further so that the process of 'getting around' is substituted and limited to the matter of using or not using a stick.

In this instance, Mrs Mitchell had already told the staff nurse that she had a home help once a week, but otherwise managed herself. The staff nurse also 'knew' the patient was out at the shop that morning where she collapsed. She had also been informed by the patient that a previous stroke affected the patient's left foot. However, what the staff nurse did not establish was whether the patient has fallen before or whether she experienced any difficulty in getting around. The nurse implies that 'using a stick' is representative of 'not being fully mobile'. All that can be said after this line of questioning is that the patient does get out and about and that she does not use a stick, but the nurse had not seen the patient walking at this point. In fact, I observed that the patient was very nimble when she did get out of bed and walk around.

Sometimes nurses shaped a patient's reply by qualifying their question and it was very rare for nurses to use completely open, undirected questions. When they did they often 'took it away' again by qualifying the question with another one.

> **Student nurse:** How's your skin? Do you get eczema, dry patches or any thing like that?
> **Mrs Appleton:** No. Just old and wrinkled.

These approaches to questioning patients about themselves appear to be a quick check on aspects of a patient which might need a nursing response. They help situate the patient in the nurses' routines. But this approach also communicates something else to patients, which is that patients' needs are not ascertained through their encounters with nurses. This process depends upon the nurses excluding any possibility that a patient's meanings help author their needs. The following extract exemplifies the method.

> **Student nurse:** Do you sleep okay? Or do you have to take any medicines?
> **Mrs Violet:** Oh no, as I said, I am up every two hours. It's just a reaction since my husband died. I wouldn't take anything. I don't like sleeping pills or anything like that – I don't believe in them.
> **Student nurse:** Do you smoke or drink at all?
> **Mrs Violet:** No, neither.
> **Student nurse:** You don't suffer from depression at all or anything like that?
> **Mrs Violet:** Oh no, I've learnt to live.

Mrs Violet had already told the nurse about the water tablets she was on and that she had to get up every two hours at night to go to the lavatory. She had repeated her statement that she got up to go to the lavatory at night when asked 'do you have any bladder problems?' In the sequence of her questions the nurse, as was usual, followed the sequence on the patient profile form, which she filled in as follows:

> **Sleep:** wakes every two hours to go to the loo
> **Occupation:** retired
> **Social activities:** doesn't smoke or drink
> **Emotional status:** good

But there is some ambiguity in Mrs Violet's replies. In her account, Mrs Violet associates waking up with both her bereavement and with a problem caused by the water tablets she is on. Mrs Violet's account implies that there may even have been some connection between the two – her heart problems (she was in hospital for this) may have arisen since the death of her husband, which led to her taking diuretic therapy. However, the nurse makes it clear that she is not going to explore the ambiguity. Her question 'you don't suffer from depression at all or anything like that?' is closed and announces that she is not probing, even indirectly, about the possibility of a disturbed emotional or mental state.

Mrs Violet, in her interview with me, said that her husband had died of a heart condition in the ward below the one she was admitted to. This was not, as far as I know, ever revealed by the nurses. When telling me about her husband the patient wept and impressed me with how distressed she was while having maintained enormous control over herself during her stay in the ward. In my dealings with her I learnt that her emotional status was a complex achievement on her behalf. She had indeed 'learnt to live'. This was a patient with a heart condition so uncovering any emotional disturbance may (or may not) have been helpful in nursing her back to health.

There are several features of the interviews which need to be emphasised. First, the sequence of the profile is used to move patients on and away from discussion. Second, the nurses' approach implies a separation of one category from another, whereas for patients there are connections. 'Weight' is connected to diet, 'sleep' is connected to 'bladder' or to emotion. Third, the terms used by the nurses are not everyday terms but are more or less 'medicalised' and, in talking with patients, the nurses frequently maintained the medical translation. In these ways there is not only a separation of different aspects, which in everyday life may be considered connected, but there is also a translation of these aspects which fragments and reduces. For example, 'bladder', 'diet' and 'bowel' are not aspects of life processes, eating and drinking and going to the lavatory, but are treated as separate entities translated into a specialist, discursive space. These methods set up discord between nurses and patients and restrict patients' responses.

During the study, nurses were not seen to discuss with patients what had brought them to hospital, their usual health or their diagnosis in any detail at any time. This may be because of the perceived 'danger' of discussing what is wrong with the patient. It must be stressed that it was not simply junior or student nurses who would not discuss these matters with patients; the senior nurses also avoided these types of discussion. As already indicated in earlier chapters, however, qualified nurses were quite happy to discuss these matters between themselves. So, while the nurse in charge at the time of the patient's admission usually came to see the patient some time soon after their arrival, any inquiry as to what had brought the

patient to hospital or how they were currently feeling appeared perfunctory (see Sister's conversation with Mrs Weston in Chapter 4 as an
example), or as a cross-check on some already known or identified issue.
In their encounters with patients around the admission period nurses
actually seemed to avoid engaging with patients to explore their experience and the meanings that the situation has for them. A patient's 'condition' was, in this way, re-presented through voices other than their own.

This did not just happen in relation to the immediate issue of diagnosing
patients, but also in relation to their usual health and to any specific issues
which could be constituted as their response to their current illness. The
nurses systematically and consistently blocked patients' participation in
the constitution of the story about them.

Disciplining patients, disciplining nurses

Nurses' methods help them to accomplish first class medicine and the
production of the clinical domain. In their encounters with patients nurses
achieve sequestration of patients' experiences and concerns. These
experiences and concerns are not only rendered insignificant but they also
cannot legitimate action and patients have no authority. Nurses' conduct
on these occasions constitutes a particular methodological approach – it
simulates a form of history and examination based upon a positivistic
science. It also reduces the patient to traits and parts. But most importantly
in relation to notions of nursing theory in which the bedside is figured as a
site of negotiation, the nurses' conduct ensures that relationships in the
clinical domain between staff and patients are non-participative – patients
are not to be included in the organisation of meaning or the production of
signs.

The overall effect is to exclude the patient from participation in the
interpretation of their condition. One knock-on effect of this, as has been
demonstrated in this chapter, is that nurses' records and their conversations about patients do not coincide with how patients see or account for
themselves (see the interview with Mrs Violet in the previous section). The
patient's voice is excluded from helping to constitute the context in which
they are viewed and in which they become visible. There is an attempt to
silence patients. But nurses are accomplishing more than this in these
encounters. They are also helping to initiate patients into the acute medical
domain where the order of knowledge rests on an idea that only some
people are disciplined enough to know. Anything which is known which
falls outside the field of the medical gaze is quite simply not worth
knowing or has to be kept backstage.

Forms of order are established by nurses through displacement and sequestration of patients' concerns and the deferral to authorities located beyond the bedside. These effects are now explored in the admission of Major Stevenson, an 80-year-old gentleman who had just arrived on the ward from A&E. According to the information sent with the patient from A&E, he probably had a urinary tract infection. He had high fevers with rigors.

[Major Stevenson is in bed, lying fairly flat. A student nurse goes to the side of the patient, carrying forms. She places these on the top of the bedside cabinet and leans on this to write. She turns to the patient and looks down when she speaks to him. She is standing above him, not close.]

Major Stevenson: If you could – I am not sure if I have any money – but if you could phone my wife?

Student nurse: Right, what is the number?

Major Stevenson: What?

Student nurse: What is the 'phone number?

Major Stevenson: Oh yes. It's [he says the phone number]. Tell her they've made a decision to keep me in hospital, ward 10.

Student nurse: Right, can I ask you a few questions first?

Major Stevenson: Yes, certainly.

[I note that the patient's mouth is terribly dry. He looks quite sallow and unwell.]

Student nurse: What's your address, please? [Major Stevenson gives it.]

Student nurse: And what's your date of birth, please? [Again, he gives the details.]

The materiality of the nursing assessment forms gives the nurse access to Major Stevenson. They are legitimated through their association with bureaucratic authority. She has papers to fill in, their formality acts as a demand (on both her and the patient). They are to be inscribed, so questions must be asked, and acts undertaken.

Major Stevenson, at the beginning of the encounter, attempts to assert his own concerns. He asks the nurse to telephone his wife, and gives precise instructions as to what she is to be told. The nurse receives the instruction, but defers it until later and she asserts that her work of asking questions is to come first. This deferral is critical and constitutes an important displacement effect. The interview continues:

Student nurse: Right, do you know why you were admitted?

Major Stevenson: I'm not quite sure – I had these pains, and shaking yesterday.

Student nurse: Do you take any medicines at all?

Major Stevenson: They're all in there [points to plastic shopping bag on bed-table. Student Nurse fetches bag and gives it to him. He takes out the tablets and reads off the labels to her. It takes quite a time].

Student nurse: How are you on your feet – any problems?

Major Stevenson: Not really, OK, I get around.

Student nurse: Do you use a stick at all?

Major Stevenson: Oh, yes.

Student nurse: How tall are you?

Major Stevenson: About five foot five and half.

Student nurse: And what weight are you?

Major Stevenson: About 9 stone.

Student nurse: Do you have any problems with your bladder?

Major Stevenson: I'm always on the run [smiles].

Student nurse: But that's because of your frusemide, isn't it [not a question]. How about your bowels?

Major Stevenson: I was a bit – so I took two pills night before last.

Student nurse: Were you constipated?

Major Stevenson: I think so.

Student nurse: Is your diet quite good?

Major Stevenson: Everything.

Student nurse: Do you suffer with dry skin at all?

Major Stevenson: Not particularly.

Student nurse: Are you allergic to anything?

Major Stevenson: Not that I am aware of.

Student nurse: Do you smoke?

Major Stevenson: I used to – I gave it up.

Student nurse: Very good.

Major Stevenson: I went to a party and came home and when I got up in the morning I smelt my clothes, it was revolting, I thought how awful for other people to smell me like that.

Student nurse: Very good. Do you ever wear glasses?

Major Stevenson: Yes.

Student nurse: Are you a good sleeper?

Major Stevenson: We go to bed at half past ten – I mean we turn out the light then. Then I wake at 12 – I take a sleeping pill then – normally, I sleep until 7.30 but if I wake up again at about 4 or 5 I take another pill.

Student nurse: Do you have any activities – what hobbies have you got?

Major Stevenson: None now. I used to do a great deal of walking, up into the Moorlands and up North – can't do it now.

Student nurse: Do you have any social workers or home helps?

Major Stevenson: No, we employ.

Student nurse: How often?

Major Stevenson: Monday and today – she came in to do the ironing.

Because my wife's like me – heart trouble. [The student nurse writes some notes.]

Now Major Stevenson is quite ill, yet the questioning is relentless. Why?

The interview can be seen as a series of moves which imply that Major Stevenson's meanings, his life-world and his experience of illness are subordinate to, or are set apart as being extraneous to, the main work of the setting. For example, he states that while he is unsure as to why he has been admitted, what brought him to the hospital were 'pains and shaking'. These, as aspects of 'how he was', are not developed by the nurse to know 'how he is now'. Further, he mentions that he suffers with 'heart trouble' but how this affects him is not pursued. Unlike in an ordinary conversation, the nurse does not pursue many leads, even over those matters such as his heart condition or his shaking and rigors which may be relevant to understanding Major Stevenson's acute condition and his current needs.

The purpose of the nurse's questions remains hidden from Major Stevenson (and quite possibly from the nurse). She does not permit him to participate in the authorisation of significance: signification and interpretation occur through orders instigated at a distance from the interaction. Neither she nor he is their author. These moves constitute the second form of displacement effect.

Towards the end of the admission Major Stevenson breaks in again, and asks for a drink:

Student nurse: I'll just do your blood pressure and pulse.
Major Stevenson: I would like a drink of some kind.
Student nurse: I'm sorry?
Major Stevenson: I would like a drink of some kind. I'm very dry.
Student nurse: Right. [She continues to write. She turns to the patient holding a wristlet name band.] I need to put this band on to tell who you are and your date of birth. And I'll check with the doctor if it's all right for you to have something to drink. [She puts the name band on.]
Major Stevenson: Oh, yes.
Student nurse: I'll just cut that end off.
Major Stevenson: Thank you. [The student nurse turns to go.]

Approximately one and half hours after the admission has been completed the patient is given a drink and is told by both the doctor and the Staff Nurse that he must drink as much as possible.

In an echo of the beginning of the interview when Major Stevenson makes a request the nurse indicates she did not hear his request for a drink, so Major Stevenson repeats the request. But now there is a critical difference: at the beginning of the encounter he did not justify his request for his wife to be informed of his admission, but he does justify his request for a drink. The earlier deferral of his request, a deferral to orders other than his own, and the following procedure appear to have produced an effect. His justification for wanting a drink, that he is very dry, indicates how he is now ready to explain himself – it has set up a justificatory context. The nurse once again defers Major Stevenson's request. First, she puts the name band on and then she establishes a new aspect of the order of things by saying that Major Stevenson, like her, 'needs' permission from a doctor before he can have a drink. This hierarchy helps her and Major Stevenson to rank his wants and to relay to Major Stevenson how he may now require permission from the nurse. It helps to establish the relationship of power and the hierarchies in the setting. Major Stevenson's thirst has no legitimacy *as a need* to which she should respond, a drink requires authorisation from someone or something else. Finally, she drives the message home by finishing her task before leaving to ask about the drink.

It is not that Major Stevenson is not being permitted to speak, but there is a problem over his authority. His attempts to authorise his own needs, as thirsty or as concerned for his wife, have an effect in that the nurse does respond. But the effect is to occasion a move, through which he is displaced. He is being moved to defer to other authorities and other orders, through which his concerns (his thirst, his wife) are either temporarily deferred or require legitimation.

The nurse's conduct certainly relays to Major Stevenson the order of things and helps accomplish the institution of a particular relationship between him and the medical practitioners. But it can be interpreted as doing more than this. The critical moment is how Major Stevenson is turned: he is turned from taking it for granted, as someone who is unwell and incapacitated, that his wants and his concerns, expressed plainly by him, will be 'taken on trust', especially by a nurse. By the end of the encounter he is compelled to give an account of himself, to justify his breaking in on the nurse's agenda and the nurse's time. ('I would like something to drink. I am very dry.') Major Stevenson is able to respond, he is able to read the instruction and acquiesce, he is able to fall into line, to learn how to be patient and, critically, how to 'do' (Garfinkel, 1967) patient. We learn from this encounter that the space between the patient and the nurse can never be constituted as a space of discretion.

The admission procedure, especially the form-filling, accomplishes something apart from acting on the patient. Like the nursing handover and the written reports, it also acts on the nurse and both reveals and affects her disciplined behaviour. As it makes something about her visible to others, so the procedure also exercises her and makes her work. Through her treating Major Stevenson as fractured, rendered to parts and traits, and in treating the admission as revealing matters of fact, a discursive space is created in which she can think of him as fractured and herself as ordering the world in particular ways. But this is not because she has discretion, as an individual. Instead, her authority comes from her participation in a discipline, a disciplined gaze.

Discussion

This chapter has mainly examined nurse–patient encounters at the time of patients' admission to hospital. Nurses interview patients in a way which mimics a medical history. This is important because the way in which the admission is performed helps to make the nurses' conduct visible as rational and important work. The forms and the ways in which they are operationalised are nurses' props, to help them dramatise their work and make it visibly official and purposeful. Nurses deploy the nursing profile form to legitimate their survey of a patient's social and functional life, but this survey reduces aspects of patients to traits and parts – it *technologises* the social.

Through these encounters a particular form of nurse–patient relationship is developed. The patient has become the object of a nursing gaze, so the nurse conducts the admission as if she is looking according to a grid of perceptions and then noting according to a code. But this conduct relays that neither the nurse nor the patient is a source of signification or legitimation; indeed, authority lies far from the bedside. This means that, in complete contrast to calls from theories of nursing, neither nurses nor patients author patients' needs. On the contrary, the admission period is a time of initiation through which nurses' conduct relays to patients that the bedside cannot be a space of discretion. Authority and legitimation lie elsewhere in other disciplined bodies of knowledge.

Through their conduct, nurses organise their relationships with patients to sustain the social organisation of the acute medical domain. This organisation accomplishes the dual agenda of first class medicine and the politics of the waiting lists. Nurses help patients to learn to efface themselves as social beings so that they can be rendered as medical objects. At the same time, nurses' conduct accomplishes a form of efficiency – they minimise the kinds of troubles that are addressed in the acute medical domain to those concerned with observation and treatment, as determined through medical discourse. Other needs, like those relating to mobility, should not be central and mobilisation should be confined to getting someone back on their feet after they begin to recover.

Through the admission period, patients learn how to conduct themselves to enable their transformation from person to patient, but not just any patient. They efface their social and personal concerns to fit the constituting of classes. To have a medical future, as we have seen in earlier chapters, a patient must have a social future and only then can they be transformed from patient back to person within a short period of time. The key feature here is that to be rendered 'appropriate' in the acute medical domain depends upon the possibility for transience. To have a medical future as a treatment space means that troubles must be reversible, and for troubles to be reversible they must not be chronic. These are the conditions for a patient to be termed 'acutely ill'. The movement from person to patient and back to person fulfils the need for visible outcomes. Only this kind of patient will do – they fit the medical agenda for a particular kind of research, as well as the new world of health care dominated by the politics of waiting lists.

In preceding chapters it has emerged that, as well as aligning with managerial and medical agendas to pull patients through the beds, nurses are also implicated in the effacement of the social and of their own contribution to medical decision making. Nurses' conduct helps patients to learn to efface the complexity of their troubles and to allow others to author their clinical needs. The question arises as to why. Why are nurses engaged in practices which appear to contradict theories of nursing? There is, of course, no simple answer. But a way of breaking up the complexity is to ask another question: what are nurses accomplishing by their alignment with the clinical domain and the effacement of the social?

This question is addressed in the following chapter where nurses' own understandings of their conduct are examined.

Chapter 6
Assessing Patients' Needs

Introduction

This chapter elaborates the idea of a nursing gaze.

So far we have focused on how nurses, together with doctors and others, organise and produce ward life. Medicine has emerged as a resource which requires distribution, and as a practice in which both nurses and doctors engage. Medicine is thus distributed in both senses but the criteria for distribution are complex. At one level, nurses and doctors make it appear that medicine is contained within purely clinical grounds. However, it seems that the alignment of managerial and medical agendas has put a greater emphasis on pulling patients through the beds, and under these conditions not all patients will do, nor are all practices acceptable.

Distribution, then, rests upon a constituting of classes (of work, of nurses and of patients), which includes aligning what is human and personal with the social, and the social is *extruded* as non-technical. Surprisingly, nurses align themselves with these agendas, although this involves nurses in the effacement of some aspects of their own contribution to medical decision making. It seems therefore that they are complicit in hiding how medicine is distributed.

This chapter examines nurses' accounts. Examining these makes visible not just how nurses think and work, but also suggests what it is that makes up a good and valuable hospital from their perspective. While nurses, like doctors, draw on medical discourse as the key method for making sense of a patient's troubles and of legitimising their own activities, they have extended the medical gaze. Indeed, in making their assessments of patients' needs, nurses go far beyond drawing on biomedical understandings.

Nurses aim to become proficient at reading patients' social histories and observing their behaviour, to contextualise their troubles as well as monitor their progress. Nurses draw upon an extraordinary range of discursive grounds upon which to make sense of what they do and what patients need. The chapter is broken down into six sections covering different aspects of how nurses ground their assessments of patients. These grounds are 'medical condition', 'age', 'context', 'lifestyle' and 'social situation', 'capability' (past and present), and 'quality of life'.

Paradoxically, nurses themselves order these matters in a hierarchy. For example, they emphasise the need to bring quality of life into play only when a patient's medical future is in doubt. So, at the same time as it becomes clear that nurses draw upon much more than biomedical knowledge to 'know' what patients need, they are also complicit in rendering these other grounds as supplementary, not complementary, to the key work of the medical domain, the performance of first class medicine and the treatment of the acutely ill. Further, and perhaps critically, nurses describe their knowing in ways which occupy the same epistemological domain as that of medicine – a nursing gaze emerges which focuses on patients not simply as a treatment space, but as a space of rehabilitation. Through their discourses nurses reveal how other kinds of epistemological ground are too weak to be persuasive or to have influence. Thus, while nurses emerge as magpies, borrowing from many disciplines, they adhere to a particular form of rationalism.

Diagnosis: placing patients in the nurses' world

At one level it is simple. Knowing what is 'wrong with patients' appears to be critical to knowing what patients need. The nurses talked about what was wrong with a patient in terms of knowing their diagnosis, what their signs and symptoms were and what treatments or investigations they were to have. Diagnosis–symptoms–treatment act to situate a patient in the nurses' world.

For example, a diagnosis of myocardial infarction implies a particular set of relationships which are taken into account by nurses in the ways they nurse those patients. These include the relationship between a clot in an artery and damaged heart muscle – to enable the heart muscle to cope and heal, the nurses maintain the patient on bed rest. Further, in expectation that the heart muscle may be compromised nurses take readings of blood pressure and pulse and observe the patient for signs such as breathlessness, chest pain or an altered fluid balance. These are the ways in which nurses translate the patient through medical discourse into a particular set of nursing responses. In this way, a diagnosis can stand for a set of nursing responses, but translation is never completely routinised.

In Chapter 2, it was shown that this way of 'knowing what to do for patients' was very much borne out by the way the nurses structured their handovers. During these, the nurses did not usually give much detailed instruction about nursing care, but rather gave information regarding the patient's medical condition and any technical details. Nursing care was frequently given in summary or in global terms such as 'all two-hourly care', or 'self-caring'. Thus, the indicators to how an individual should be nursed were carried in the details of the patient's medical condition but, as discussed in the previous chapter, this was not a knee-jerk response. The nurses spent time analysing what they saw and what the doctors did for patients to know what a patient needed, at the same time maintaining an undecidedness over precisely what was wrong with the patient. In other words, the nurses continuously assessed and reviewed a patient's situation.

This routinised approach obviates the requirement for doctors' orders except in specific cases. However, it also relies on a nurse's ability to read the medical discourse on patients to extract the relevant issues and, further, to know what contingencies necessitate or suggest a deviation, and when permission should be sought. For example:

> **Staff nurse:** So we have a sort of format, but we do bend it. It is pliable depending on the patient. That is usually decided by the doctors.
> **Researcher:** What, whether or not you get cracking?
> **Staff nurse:** Yes, we would actually be reluctant to start somebody mobilising early without permission, and that would be decided on the doctors' rounds usually – 'we have to get this woman moving, start mobilising her'.

Routinised responses are nurses' frames of reference for their practices (see also Berg, 1992). Deviations from the routine necessitate justification, such as special permission from the doctors. For example, while nurses themselves sometimes said that doctors' permission had to be sought in order to deviate from routines, these accounts also illustrate that nurses decided *how* they want to deviate, *then* they got the permission. This practice shows how adept nurses could be at playing the system, to shift accountability for decisions onto medical staff.

The degree to which the relationship is explicitly routinised between medical condition and nursing response varies. In the study, for patients with possible heart attack (myocardial infarction) there was an explicit protocol. This was pinned up on the wall at the nurses' station but it only referred to the mobilisation aspects of patients and the giving of an information booklet to patients close to their discharge. The nurses kept using this in their hypothetical examples throughout their interviews. However, in many respects, there was a far less explicit relationship between a patient's condition and nursing care. In these circumstances nurses needed information about the patient in terms of their signs, symptoms and provisional diagnoses. So, while the nurses presented themselves as reliable and confident in their translation of medical issues into nursing care they in turn relied upon being kept informed by doctors about these medical issues. This put them into a dependent relationship with doctors – nurses rely on being kept informed by doctors. Some nurses in the study said that doctors seemed to make access to information difficult.

In summary, nurses interpret and translate their own observations of patients, as well as the medical talk and notes about patients, into nursing care. Some are routinised responses, some responses are instituted as protocols, while more often than not the medical picture is unclear and nurses engage in interpretative work. Nurses do not usually require instructions from medical staff and 'know' the responses and routines; problems arise when doctors do not keep nurses informed and up-to-date. Last, deviations from the routines may require an explicit justification, including permission from medical staff.

But medical discourse is just one of the ciphers which allow nurses to translate a patient's troubles into forms of care. Other aspects of a patient's situation mediate and even transform interpretation and translation of the medical talk about a patient. In particular, the nurses assess the future by laying a patient's past alongside their medical present.

Capability

The nurses in the study referred to how they needed to know about a patient's 'social situation'. Other ways of referring to this social situation were 'home life', 'context' and 'lifestyle'. The survey of a patient's social and functional life is called 'getting a history'. In a history a patient's 'home' or 'social' situation was connected to family support, usual ability to 'self-care', mobility, and community services (either health or social). Taken together these aspects indicated how capable a patient was on a normal basis.

Getting a 'history' has different uses. First, knowing about a patient's normal mobility or ability to self-care enables comparison with the present to know what is abnormal. Some of the nurses in the study claimed that knowing what someone was like normally gave them something to aim for in their rehabilitation of patients – a history gives you a 'goal'. In the following extract, a staff nurse is talking about a patient she admitted the previous day. This patient had been described by A&E staff as a 'total wreck' with a 'knackered heart'.

> Staff nurse: ...so in that case we were able to see she was capable of quite a lot. Already we could assess that she was capable of doing a lot for herself. I spoke to the patient, I spoke to her daughter, and I got a

clear picture in my mind and then wrote up the care plan according to what I thought her needs were from there.

JL: So what sort of things did you get from them?

Staff nurse: Basically a history of what has happened over the past few days, for a start, leading up to the admission, so the recent history was about what led up to the admission. A history of what she was like before she took ill this time, so that at least for the long term this means you know what you're trying to get the patient back to.

JL: You got a base to . . . ?

Staff nurse: You've got a baseline picture. Now, I know that up until Sunday this woman was totally self-caring, so if we were thinking now in the long term we're trying to get this patient back to that, to that level. Up until Sunday she was totally looking after herself.

The staff nurse stresses how knowing about the patient in terms of her past capability acts as a 'baseline picture'. A baseline is important in terms of being able to aim for something. The nurse's metaphors, 'baseline' and 'level', imply that the past acts as an objective measurement against which to judge the patient's rehabilitation. However, the staff nurse also implies that she is going to nurse the patient in the present in a different way because 'up until Sunday this woman was totally self-caring', she was 'totally looking after herself'. It suggests that she is going to nurse this woman in a way appropriate to someone who is normally totally self-caring, rather than nurse them as someone who has been totally dependent for the last few years. Tacitly, the past has transformed the present by offering the possibility of a future. The preoccupation with self-care has been described by Rudge (1997), drawing on Rafferty (1996), as a nursing hegemony.

Some nurses in the study spoke in terms of 'goodness' in relation to capability – through this realism there can be optimism (something to work for). What is emerging is that, for the nurses, there was a similar notion underpinning their assessment practices to that which underpinned the medical staff's need for a patient to provide a treatment space. I would like to refer to this as a 'space of rehabilitation'. A patient was assessed in relation to whether or not they would provide both a treatment space and a space for progress and movement, up a hierarchical set of conditions. This means that a patient had to be available to the nurses as a project of recovery.

For example, one staff nurse talked explicitly about 'levels', about moving from total chaos up to something better. This seemed to be measured in terms of the patient's capability and was related to 'goodness'. Being 'capable' and being 'knackered' or a 'total wreck' are juxtaposed and act as indicators of the good, or presumably its opposite, 'chaos', which is 'bad'. In some way knowing about a patient in terms of their previous preadmission state gave the nurse a sense of their worth. Strathern (1997) helps elucidate how Euro-Western thought proceeds by drawing relations of comparison.

A history is important in a second way because it alerted the nurses to possible problems with getting a patient home. A history can indicate breakdown in an older person's life, which in turn led to the nurses realising that they needed to send out into the community to 'look' for further evidence of this person's capability. The following extract illustrates this.

> **Sister:** I think it is very important especially with a view to them going back. If they've come in having collapsed at home and are unable to cope at home you don't want to send them back into the same situation without any help, for them to bounce back into hospital within two or three days. You need to know whether they've got home helps, meals on wheels, a district nurse, a hospital club, day hospitals or social clubs that they go to. Usually, if their relatives are staying with them, we need to know if their relatives are prepared to look after them for a little while after they come out of hospital, or if the relatives are prepared to put a bit more input into them when they are discharged? You need to know quite a lot about a patient, you need to know whether they live upstairs in a flat, you need to know whether they're on a ground floor.

Sister emphasises how it is important to know about a patient's social situation and their family life 'with a view to them going back'. The implication is that a patient may be in hospital because of their situation: 'you don't want to send them home into the same situation without any help, for them to bounce back into hospital'. Sister envisages 'social situation' in terms of support to enable 'coping', and relates this to discharge arrangements, which are important matters with respect to older or disabled patients.

From their conversation it appeared that most of the nurses in the study only regarded a history as important where there was potential for or an actual problem in a patient's 'social situation'. Specifically, this was in terms of a patient's 'capability', that is their mobility and their 'self-care' ability and how this is balanced against the support they need and can get. A history was considered really only necessary for older or disabled people, as the following extract indicates:

> **Sister:** You certainly wouldn't ask a 19-year-old who's come in having had pneumonia if they have a home help or district nurse or health visitor because you assume that before they came in they were quite able

to look after themselves. But the elderly, on the other hand, they do need a lot of social support.

A third way in which a history is important is because it can permit a deviation from normal protocols. Once again this is mainly in the context of nursing older people:

> **Staff nurse:** Then having said that, it (the protocol for patients with myocardial infarction) is sometimes changed. For example, if it was an 85-year-old lady who obviously needs to be kept mobile, if we immobilise her too much as we would do initially for a post MI then that is going to be worse for her because she's going to become totally immobile. You know, she needs to walk, she's got arthritis, she's got a history of DVT [deep vein thrombosis], whatever. We need this woman walking so we might walk her quicker than we would somebody else.

For this staff nurse, the past medical history (a history of DVT) and present secondary diagnosis (arthritis), coupled with the patient's age, modify her usual response to translating a diagnosis of MI into nursing care which would usually be bed rest or restricted mobility. Her example is informative as it once again focuses on how older patients may require a different response, instituting deviations from the usual routine response to the primary medical condition. Once again, it is in terms of mobility that the past is raised. Histories help nurses maintain the flow.

Finally, there is a fourth way in which a history can support nurses' work of knowing what a patient needs. This explanation for why history is important only emerged on one occasion during the study. Knowing about a patient in terms of their background can inform decisions about care, by enabling understanding about a person's current experience. The following extract illustrates this.

> **Staff nurse:** I was particularly frustrated in one patient's case, because we had quite a quiet evening shift that night and she was upset when we settled her down. I sat with her for about half an hour, just holding her hand and talking to her and asking her why she was crying, and all the rest of it. One of the students sat with her for half an hour and we actually said afterwards that, you know, it's that she's 95, she's never been away from home before, she's scared, and I was trying to get across that sometimes in the elderly all this external stimulus, all the noise of the ward, the change in your team, everything can make them go as if they're really confused.

In this extract the staff nurse is saying that background information about an older patient can enable better *understanding* of the present, so that judgements about requirements are contextualised. Interestingly, the case referred to involves a confused old person, someone who could no longer continue in the situation to control their own behaviour, acting out normality and concealing their distress. By implication, nurses do not need to know about the background and lifestyle of strictly 'medical' patients; it is 'added on' information in the context of older patients. Thus, knowing about patients as persons to help understand their needs in the present is itself downgraded as a further aspect of the constituting of classes.

From most of the nurses' conversations with me, it would appear that a patient's 'social situation' and their past life was important strategically to managing the future: the disposal of patients. Further, the past history of a patient may indicate the necessity for deviations from routinised responses to the medical condition ascribed to patients, where working to the usual responses might act to impede recovery and mobilisation. The staff nurse's conversation above shows how a patient's past can inform the present in terms of the interpretation of a patient's nursing requirements, and can even act to transform the interpretation of a patient's 'condition'. This in turn has revealed how nurses may estimate patients with respect to some notion of value which revolves around patients' conduct, their capability, and their motivation and ability to self-care. Thus, what emerges from the nurses' conversation is how older patients, unlike that other 'proper' class of patient, the 'acute medical patient', cannot be viewed simply in relation to their ascribed medical condition.

Nurses enrol aspects of a patient's social situation to extend the scope of their gaze and enable an assessment of patients in relation to their future and their potential as a space of rehabilitation. This extension to patients' psychosocial and emotional life does not seem to be used to give practitioners access to more extensive grounds upon which to call patients to account (Silverman, 1987), but enables estimates of a patient's capability and potential for movement. The difficulty is that the social and age are connected. This association with the non-clinical is problematic for the identities of both older patients and nurses because, within the context of a constituting of classes, the social is polluting to the purity of the medical domain. It is, at best, supplementary and at worst, demeaning.

How age itself mediates the relationship between medical condition and the nursing response is considered in the next section.

Age

All the nurses in the study said they needed to know a patient's age in order to know how to nurse them. Explaining why raises controversial and ambivalent issues. Some of the nurses suggested that knowing a patient's age would affect their nursing care because there are specific problems, potential or actual, which older people are prone to and which require close monitoring or a nursing response. These included specific issues such as constipation, pressure sores, urinary tract infection, sensitivity to drugs, and mental and functional vulnerability to illness and admission to hospital.

However, the nurses seemed to have an ambivalence to older people. This ambivalence revolved around how attention to the 'social' dimension of illness was important to the nursing care of older people, but that the social was not an appropriate dimension on an acute medical ward. This situation incurred feelings of ambivalence and nurses felt that they were failing older people, and indeed that older people stood as a reminder of their failure to care. For example, a staff nurse described the care of the elderly on the ward as a 'shambles'. She told me that many of the nurses and doctors were very knowledgeable about older people's specific needs and that 'most nursing is looking after the elderly so we're all quite experienced at it'. However, she said that they were not giving the elderly what they needed because they could not give older people the social care they required.

Nursing activities described as social included talking, entertaining, flicking through a magazine, mental stimulation, having relationships, or taking them out. But the nurses also downplayed these kinds of activities as non-technical and inappropriate to the acute medical domain. The staff nurse said that 'being hidebound by the routine' somehow got in the way of appreciating older patients as people, which is related to their identity in the past:

> **Staff nurse:** For a lot of elderly people, especially if they can remember, what happened to them in their youth is so much more important to them than what's happening to them now. And valuing, you know, making others value them.
> **JL:** But valuing their experiences?
> **Staff nurse:** Their experiences and that they've raised families and that you're only a slip of a girl as she says before she clobbers you round the ear with her wash bowl [laughs].

The staff nurse suggests that the present is not as important to older people as their past, and that their past constitutes to a certain extent their self-identity in the present. She also suggests that it is through talking with older people that you can value them as people in the present. This notion was echoed in the accounts of other nurses in both wards. They all regretted that they could not do more for the older patients 'socially'.

None of the nurses defined the social as in any way important to a patient's medical condition.

Authentic acutely ill people require purely clinical care. Where the social intrudes upon the present there is something wrong, not with the nurses, but with the patient, who becomes less than authentic. A conversation with Sister indicates this:

> **Sister:** I find it very difficult because I honestly don't think it's the right place for an elderly person to be if they're not ill. Because they're low priority in an acute hospital, they are not given the time they need. And we tend to do that. Bay 4 is bay 4, it rarely changes. It's very basic nursing care, and basic nursing care is all they get for most of the time. The priority are the acutely ill. Whether they're young or geriatric they need more nursing time than somebody who is 91 and waiting for a long-term bed in a geriatric ward. It is certainly not ideal, although most of these ladies have come in with an acute condition and very soon after they've arrived their acute condition has resolved and they are back to their best, which is often a chronic senile dementia. And once they're in hospital you really find out how unable to cope in the community they are so you don't send them back out. And they're left to sit in an acute medical ward waiting for 18 months to 2 years for a geriatric bed.

Sister later explained at my request her distinction between the acute patient and a geriatric patient:

> **Sister:** I think loosely the term 'geriatric' is used by most people for a lot of people over the age of 65. But I find there are some geriatrics who are only 40.
> **JL:** What do you mean by that?
> **Sister:** Well it depends upon the person, there are some very young, mentally young 90-year-olds who I would never describe as being geriatric. I would say they were elderly. Geriatric, I would say, are dependent people, elderly dependent people, who need a certain amount of nursing care.
> **JL:** Physically?
> **Sister:** Physically dependent. Ladies who are confused . . .

So not all older people are 'geriatric' or 'social'.

These discourses indicate something deeply embedded in the ways in which the nurses conceive of the differences between older people and other ill people – that is, what they conceive of as acute illness. Illness is constituted by them as something medical and as detached from the social. This extends to how they conceptualise their nursing care: they constitute themselves as nurses who prioritise medical and technical aspects and who do not really operate in a social dimension, except as a luxury. And further, as has been seen in earlier sections, the social can act as a *drag* on the medical or technical. It gets in the way, to produce patients who are not medical but whose problems are 'caused' by their age and by their lack of support, and who need social care. It is also very important to note that older people are figured as having a past which is important, while their future is being figured as not so important to them.

Some of the nurses refuted the idea that age affected their nursing care. One of the Sisters and a staff nurse said that because they primarily nurse the *condition* rather than the *patient*, and that this constitutes a fair and rational way of going on, then it follows that any patient, no matter what their age, is treated by them in the same way. However, they both gave the proviso that this depended upon whether the patient's medical condition was being actively treated. The elderly 'are very much judged on their own merit' and 'should have the care that they require' given their medical condition and no matter what their age. There are differences; for example, nurses talked about patients who are 'not to be treated' or 'not for resus [resuscitation]' and for these patients nursing care would be different from that which would normally be given for a particular medical condition. There is also a notion of being treated fairly, according to the medical condition. It is regardless of age but has the future acting as a condition of possibility.

> **Sister:** Well if they [an elderly person] come in with an acute illness they are nursed as though they are, if they've an acute illness it doesn't matter how old they are. Frankly because you are always looking to get them well and home. And it doesn't matter whether you are nineteen or ninety, if *you've a prospect ahead of you* it doesn't matter how old you are, they come in, they're treated and they go home. [emphasis added]

Sister says 'if you've a prospect ahead of you' then you will be treated fairly and squarely, and the nurses adjust their care on that basis.

With age comes a difference in the treatment of patients which is dependent upon the assessment of a patient's future prospects. But these differences are very carefully assessed and nurses are at pains to ground their assessments in objective methods. How nurses define their own objectivity in order to assess the future is now discussed.

'Just by looking'

The nurses in the study talked about getting to know about patients in terms of what was *visible*. 'Looking' at patients should be understood as having both a literal and virtual meaning for the nurses. There was constant reference to knowing aspects of patients' requirements in terms of 'seeing', 'looking' and 'getting a picture'. While it is recognised here that in everyday language 'seeing' and 'looking' are used as dead metaphors, in the present context, 'looking' as method for the nurses had a deeper significance.

A staff nurse said that her initial way of finding out how a patient was would be to 'look at her'. She said that she could tell 'just by looking at them if they're in pain', but that she would then cross-check by asking how they were. She also claimed that, on doctors' ward rounds, she could 'tell just by looking at the patient if they're confused by what they've [the doctors] said, if they're anxious or whatever', so that she would know to return to the patient afterwards and help elucidate what the doctors said. This nurse was claiming here that she could understand some of the patients' requirements, some of what is going on inside, by reading their behaviour through looking. She was prepared to cross-check her reading of the situation by asking the patient, but the emphasis for her was on seeing for herself and reading what she saw as the visible signs of the patient's experience. In her examples, 'pain' and 'confusion' are manifested in behaviour. An aspect of the nurse's 'look' is an appraisal of the patient – summing up how they are. In the following extract, a staff nurse talks about how she knows what people need from her:

Staff nurse 1: Well, I think you can just assess a lot of people very quickly when they come in, just by the way they act. Usually, it's easy to spot if someone's really anxious when they first come in . . .

The staff nurse is making the claim that she can assess 'a lot of people' quickly when they come in 'just by the way they act'. For example, knowing that a patient is anxious can be seen by the way they act and it is easy to spot. For this nurse, knowing whether or not a patient is anxious was important and, as she said later, she believed that people can get into 'such a state that they can actually exacerbate their illness'. She also said that if patient had chest pain and was really anxious she would then need to 'keep a special eye on them'.

The nurses talk in terms of a way of seeing, which is informed and judgmental. The word 'act', used by the staff nurse, may refer to the observable manifestations of anxiety in a patient's behaviour, such as the arrangement of their face and hands and their eye movements, that is, their 'body language'. The word 'act' may also include the speech dimension, so-called 'speech acts'. But the staff nurse is describing her method of knowing only in terms of seeing, in terms of what is visible.

The staff nurse went on in her interview to contrast 'spotting' with a situation where a patient is in some way not themselves, not able to act themselves, that is when they are 'confused' or 'clapped out'. The staff nurse said that it is important to know how a patient was 'usually' but that certain conditions dis-enabled the patient from 'act'-ing as they 'usually' were. In this situation she was unable to 'see' them 'act' their normal self. In this instance, 'you' ask someone else who knows the patient, what they are 'usually like'. The staff nurse said that she got to know about how patients 'usually' were through talk. But talk in her mind was converted or translated into an image, into the visible: she used talk to help 'build' up a 'picture' of someone over time. Although this phrase is resonant with the phrase 'the mind's eye', it implies translating what becomes known, through talking with relatives, into thinking as if it has been observed, thinking talk as visible. So, for this staff nurse, even what goes on inside a person – their feelings and experience of the present – is somehow observable, knowable by seeing.

Staff nurse 2 talked about 'looking' for herself when she was worried about a particular aspect of a patient's condition she wanted to be 'observed', such as pressure areas. Seeing for herself here is related to 'knowing for sure'. This nurse felt that only by seeing for herself could she be sure of something. She also discussed how 'looking' on the morning drug round enabled her to do a crude assessment of how patients were:

> **Staff nurse 2:** Oh well it's just general, I mean, anybody who is looking very breathless or is looking as though they are in pain. It's just basic, crude observations, you know, that you have a person with a left ventricular and you've just been told their weight's up and you notice they're sitting gasping for breath. You think, 'I'll get something done about this, see about you later'. Just very crude, not all the ins and outs of how, what they've been thinking about overnight, just a crude assessment.

Here, the staff nurse uses the word 'looking' (like something) with respect to the patient, so that she can 'observe' their problem. She announces that this is 'just basic, crude observations' and contrasts it with what presumably she thinks of as less crude assessment: 'all the ins and outs, what they've been thinking about overnight'. She implies that previous information given to her, relating to the patient's diagnosis and their current condition ('left ventricular failure' and 'their weight is up'), directs or gives meaning to what she is seeing, transforming 'seeing' into the technical expertise of 'observation'. Medical discourse makes visible what she is looking at. A patient 'gasping for breath' contains both *auditory* ('gasping' as the sound of laboured intake of breath) and *visual* ('gasping' with the mouth gaping open and with chest heaving up and down) information about a patient.

However, for staff nurse 2, both are visible evidence, observations which support the facts about the patient, that the patient has heart failure and that their weight is up. Another staff nurse also explained later how they 'observe' fluid intake and output and weigh all patients on diuretics daily so that they can 'see' if the patient is 'actually passing urine'. Not passing urine or losing weight would signify heart failure.

It should be noted that staff nurse 2 takes the evidence as meaning that she needs to do something about the patient's condition 'later'. She does not give any indication of how she translates what she sees into how the patient may be feeling about their situation or into some kind of nursing discourse about how she can act directly toward the patient (for example, find out how the patient is feeling, make sure she is sitting up or well supported, check if her mouth is dry, give her a sip of water, comfort her if she is afraid). These bedside nursing aspects do not enter the nurse's picture. She is not an embodied presence, understanding through proximity to her patient. As with the nursing handover, the specific nursing response is taken for granted.

The nurses' representations of their assessments are 'clinical'. They present themselves as cognitive subjects who look at patients with a disciplined gaze. But, as already indicated, the point of reference is not how the patient is feeling, or comfort and relief of suffering, but how capable the patient is, whether or not they are recovering or whether they need more or a different treatment. Nurses are caught in, and reproduce, the endless relationship between positive knowledge, seeing and saying.

Nurses mentioned over and over during the study that they do not have time to talk, but that they use conversation as a check on their observations of patients. In this way, talk is the supplement to sight. In the next section I discuss how nurses use talk, not to know, but to help facilitate patients' recovery through the disposal of feelings.

Talking with patients: persuasion and the disposal of feelings

The purpose of talking with patients was described variously by nurses during the study. What is interesting is that nurses rarely mentioned 'listening' to patients in their interviews. Conversation with patients was characterised as 'chat' and as method. Talk as method was applied by different nurses to different situations: reassuring, cross-checking how a patient was, getting information about how a patient usually was (their 'history'), explanation, socialising and valuing[1]. Most nurses stressed that they did not have time to talk, and that they did not use talk to know what patients needed. But they did emphasise how they used talk as a cross-check on their observations. The question arises as to when the nurses prioritise talk with patients: when does it become a necessity?

In the nurses' accounts a patient's need to talk often stemmed from their need for information, explanation or reassurance. For example, in her interview one of the Sisters said that she thought that patients felt 'neglected' because they did not usually get a chance to talk about what it was that was worrying them until it was long past:

Sister: Generally we just don't talk to patients. We carry out our work procedures, you know, bathing, feeding, washing, dressing, and that's basically all they get when there are five or six people on. It's nice when there are more staff on, then the patients don't feel so neglected.
JL: Do you think they actually feel neglected?
Sister: I'm sure they do. I'm sure they, the ladies there. Constantly they say, 'Nurse, nurse, Sister can you come and speak to me?' and you say 'I'll be there in a minute'. Now when you do that to a patient you do try and get back within five or ten minutes but very often you don't. Very often towards the end of a shift you think, 'My God, Mrs So and So wanted to speak to me, I better go and see her' and by that time she has got over whatever crisis she was going through and she didn't really need you then. But when there are enough staff on, I find I can go and quite happily chat to anybody.

Sister reveals her priorities and the meaning that talking with patients has for her. Talking with patients is something separate from her ongoing activities, which take priority over talking. She does not count all the activity around a patient as a kind of language of care, nor does she mention talking with patients when administering to the body – when giving a bed bath, for example. She constitutes talking with patients as something separate from the mainstream of caring for patients, and further, she characterises talk as something the patient needs to do rather than as something she needs to do to help her know about her patients. Talk is associated with a 'crisis' or a patient's 'worry' and as extraneous to any assessment of central nursing issues. By suggesting that the patient can usually sort a problem out for themselves anyway, Sister denigrates the need for talk. The implication is that 'neglect' is not professional neglect – 'not talking' with patients does not constitute any grave impediment to delivering the goods, that is, their recovery from acute illness. Talk is something patients 'feel' the need for, and this is not really of any momentous importance because they get over whatever they wanted to talk about by the end of a shift. Unlike real medical problems, problems which require talk are transient, so they are not high on Sister's busy agenda.

For some nurses, talking is a patient need and is intimately bound up with patients *disposing* of their negative feelings. To put it simply, talk for nurses is psychological. For example, one of the Sisters gave two examples of patients to whom she did talk. She described one as a 'very inadequate young woman' with 'low self-esteem' and the other as 'introspective' with a past which she allowed to haunt her at a time when she should be worried by the present. Both were anomalies for Sister. Their need to talk was given a psychological explanation and it had nothing to do with her assessment of their nursing needs as medical patients.

In such instances nurses seemed to use talk as a method. There was a tacit understanding that anxiety and other emotions might get in the way of a smooth recovery, including compliance with treatment. So, while talk may be characterised as an interruption to everyday work, there is also a reason for allowing patients to talk as this helps prevent difficulties, such as a refusal to comply with treatment or being so worried or upset that the condition is worsened. Thus, talk is an available strategy to prevent potential blockage to the flow through the beds. But, and this is important, the patients who need talking to are constituted as having other than purely medical needs, and as such they are downgraded.

On occasion talk helps control patients through 'persuasion'. The Sisters and a staff nurse discussed how patients usually complied with the nurses' decisions about their nursing needs. They said that they would not 'force' a patient to do anything against their will. One Sister pointed out that most people were only too happy to conform, so their 'will' was in harmony with the will of the nursing staff anyway. But talk could be used to persuade as a supplement to ensure an overlap of will, and the following extract illustrates this.

> **Staff nurse:** An MI [myocardial infarction] lady wouldn't stay in her bed and was up and down and up and down. That night she was up talking with us and saying that her husband had died in CCU [Cardiac Care Unit]. Actually, I hadn't appreciated that he had died in CCU, I thought he had died at home but he had spent a lot of time in CCU. She was concerned that she was going to end up a cripple like him before his death and that she was on her own as well. But she was difficult *because she was not complying with our way that we wanted to treat her and we couldn't get it through to her* that we wanted her to stay in her bed because of her chest pain, and because we didn't know what it was. Maybe she was trying to prove to herself that 'no, this isn't going to happen to me, it can't be what my husband had' – it was maybe denial she was going through... [emphasis added]

The staff nurse is describing how the patient would not stay in bed as required by the protocol for nursing patients with heart attack. She uses talk in her attempt to achieve the patient's 'compliance'. Once again, talk enters as a tool to sort out patients with complex psychological problems but it is not being associated directly with their medical needs.

Talk was not presented by the nurses as important to knowing what patients need in the same way as getting a history or observations are. Talk emerged as supplementary, either as a cross-check with looking or as a method of persuasion. However, the nurses did not completely abandon the importance of the social as a medium for knowing patients. This comes into its own as the bottom line when the question of quality of life is raised.

Quality of life

One staff nurse said she needed to know how someone is in 'their self' in order to decide how to proceed with their nursing care. But knowing how someone is in their self is problematic.

When the nurses talked about 'knowing how someone is', they often spoke about judging a patient as an experiencing self from the outside, from the visible. They referred to knowing if someone was in pain or whether they were anxious or confused, not by what people had told them, but 'just by looking'. These aspects of a patient's situation were not seen as unimportant by the nurses, but there was a level at which they were seen as *separate* from the central focus of their activity: getting patients 'well and home'.

When some of the nurses discussed a patient whom the doctors wanted to stop treating they drew on grounds which they usually made absent. An aspect of quality medical decision making included assessing the utility of treatment. When this was in doubt, quality of life was used to inform decision making. Quality of life was partly assessed through nurses' surveillance of patients' psychosocial lives. But what the nurses emphasised was that quality of life could not be assessed through measurement alone. When it came to the bottom line (a life and death decision), quality of life could only be assessed through knowing the patient as a person. The following conversation with one of the staff nurses illustrates this. She talks about a woman, Mona, whose treatment has been discontinued.

> **Staff nurse:** It is a very difficult decision [not to treat the patient with antibiotics]. I don't feel that the medical staff were saying that she had no quality of life, but I feel that I don't think it's up to them to decide, in her case, and I think that she should have been treated.
> **JL:** When you say quality of life, you think her quality of life warrants her to continue to be treated? How do you know that?
> **Staff nurse:** Well, for a start I think she was happy enough. I think she

was quite content. Maybe you or I or one of the doctors wouldn't be happy sitting in a chair in a ward all day and probably having to go into some sort of an institution for the rest of your life, but I don't think, in her case, she would have minded that. I just feel that she should have been treated. I don't think the medical staff ever saw her as we did either. She was shouting out quite distressed yesterday and I sort of went in and asked for her to be written up for opiates, and he said, 'Oh yes, that's the first time I've heard her even speak, she's just sat there mute for six months', and I said, 'That's rubbish, she has not'. He says, 'Oh she just used to sit there and stare into space the whole time', so I said, 'Well, you don't know her very well then'.

'Quality of life' was associated by the nurse with how the patient felt about their life – 'happy enough', 'content' – and with what *that person's experience* was of their situation. The nurse said 'maybe you or I or one of the doctors wouldn't be happy … but I don't think she would have minded that'. The question is, how did the staff nurse *know* how Mona felt, or how did she think she knew? The implication is that she experienced the person 'Mona', that by being with and seeing her day-to-day, the staff nurse constructed her identity in relation to something other than medical or nursing discourse. The staff nurse's view of Mona was informed by understandings derived from a relationship of proximity (Bauman, 1990) – she has allowed Mona to have a face, to be an authority without force (Bauman, 1990, 1991; Latimer, 1997). This move is critical because in other areas of ward life the nurses do not allow patients to authorise any of the nurses' activities, including their definitions of a patient's troubles!

The staff nurse mentioned how the doctors allowed their understanding that Mona's family could not take her home to influence their decision. She went on to say that she would not allow it to influence her view:

> **Staff nurse:** I think what annoyed me more than anything else was the fact that they said they were going to stop them [the antibiotics] because she had poor home circumstances and her family couldn't take her home. I don't think you should base your criteria on whether to treat somebody or not on what sort of home circumstances they have. The way they were saying it was if she had a caring family who were willing to take her home, then they would have carried on the antibiotic treatment.

It should be noted here that this patient was 54 years old and she was in the category termed 'young chronic sick'. There is very limited provision in the community for this group, outside of placement in a long-term geriatric ward or their own home. The staff nurse felt that it was wrong to allow this aspect of a patient's situation to influence any treatment decision. Later, she mentioned that she was not 'one of these people for treating everybody, you know I wouldn't, if she was riddled with cancer or something I would be the first to agree with just letting her go'. So, for the staff nurse, knowing how to care for someone included judging a person's situation in some way on its own merits, and this is only possible if you know how that person experiences their situation by spending time with the person. This nurse said she was left feeling 'sick' that there was not more she could do for this patient.

Another staff nurse also talked about Mona:

> **Staff nurse:** Yes, because her quality of life was actually quite good. I mean I'm not one for treating people whose quality of life I feel is poor, you know, but I thought her quality of life was really okay. Maybe, what, six weeks ago, she seemed happy within herself and although she was a blocked bed, which is what they're probably thinking about, her quality of life was good, and I don't think we had the right to turn round and say you know 'tough, you've got a chest infection, tough, you're only 54 we're going to let you linger and linger and linger'.

The staff nurse saw communication with the doctors as the problem. She felt they did not *know* Mona as well as the nurses did, they had not experienced Mona the 'person', and they did not take into account the view of people who did know, the nurses.

> **Staff nurse:** Because we know Mona better. The way that they can assess quality of life from the end of the bed is different from the way that we can assess quality of life, when we see her at half ten at night sitting down in the day room having a really good chat and a joke. She's a very, very witty lady, you can enjoy her company.
> **JL:** I noticed this morning that you joked with her a lot. You mean she's a sociable person?
> **Staff nurse:** When she was better, she was one of the more sociable patients on the ward, and we had a lot of young people in. They really enjoyed her company.

The nurses felt able to judge someone's quality of life because they felt they knew a patient as a person and that this was important. The difference arises through nurses' proximity to the patients. Doctors attempt to assess quality of life 'from the end of the bed', while nurses are closer to the patients and they have experience of them in a relationship of proximity. In the relationship shown in the conversation above, the patient comes to matter as one who makes others laugh and with whom one can have a conversation.

As shown previously, it can be seen that nurses do not usually count their feelings about patients as persons as in any way relevant to their assessment of the patients. On the contrary, they pride themselves on not taking patients personally; the personal, as indicated in the handovers, only enters as a tag-on to the main focus of the assessment of a patient's medical condition and their capability ('he's a poor wee soul' or 'she's a nice lady'). The nurses are, in their discursive practices, uninterested on the whole in the individual person.

Knowing what a person's life means to them and having feelings about patients entered the nurses' discourses at the point where there was a question mark over whether the person's life was worth living or not, whether they had a prospect ahead of them, not as a treatment space with a medical future, nor as a space of rehabilitation, but as a person. Some nurses wanted to include the question of whether a patient had a *social* future as a person as the bottom line when taking medical decisions, even if treatment might in the longer term prove futile.

Discussion

Nurses' talk constitutes a nursing gaze, a grid through which patients are viewed. A nursing gaze extends the purely medical gaze. While the medical condition of the patient places a patient in the nurses' world, for a patient to be a treatment space they must also have a medical future. And nurses keep in play how a medical future depends upon whether the patient has a *social* future.

The nurses' gaze supplements the medical gaze by surveying the patient in relation to the prospect they have ahead of them. The nursing gaze is concerned with weighing up whether a patient, given all the complexity of their particular circumstances, constitutes a space of rehabilitation or not. They survey the patient's history, their psychosocial life, their conduct and their capacity to help themselves. But this is not a one-off look, it goes on over time.

Through their continuous survey, nurses evaluate whether a patient has 'a prospect ahead of them'. But when all else fails, the nurses draw upon their experience of the patient as a person: for a patient to have a medical future as a treatment space they must finally, like Mona, have a future as a person. In this, Mona differs from Jessie, discussed in Chapter 2. The problem with Jessie was that, as a person, she was no longer responding to others, no longer willing, no longer 'social'.

I have suggested that nurses ascribe patients to classes. Both their gaze, and the field of visibility which it constructs (in which nurses and patients work), are partly defined through the constituting of classes of patients. But nurses are meticulous – they hold the patient on the medical ground through drawing on many different discourses to make patients visible as persons with a prospect ahead of them. Critically, they institute this gaze as objective knowledge. Only in doing this does their extended gaze have influence, even as a supplement to the medical discourse.

In a world seeking to dispose of patients who are difficult, in terms of length of stay and in terms of demonstrating medical effectiveness, nurses have constructed a gaze which not only makes patients visible in relation to medical and nursing discourse, but which also makes visible the needs of those patients who could so easily constitute a drag on the flow. At the same time as they appear to never lose sight of the different agendas with which they feel charged (first class medicine, a professional approach to care and an efficient and equitable service), nurses' discourse is characterised by flexibility.

Their methods appear very different from the decision-making model of nursing assessment offered by technologies such as the nursing process, or from the more sentimental views of nursing which would have nurses and patients in participative and communal relations. In the harsh world of modern health services, nurses must be able to argue for patients from strong, not weak, discursive positions. Following examination of the nursing handovers and ward reports discussed in Chapter 3, patients' experiences and views hold little weight. But so does anything to do with the social. What counts is the objective world of clinical medicine. Thus, while for nurses quality of life cannot be measured, its assessment has ultimately to entail subjectivity and this makes quality of life an impossibly weak ground upon which to argue for a patient's medical future.

Nurses are compelled then to perform their knowledge practices as dependent upon visible evidence. They constitute themselves as having a disciplined gaze – in their discourse they are expert *eyes*. In the ways in which they portray their knowledge practices, these nurses are locked into an epistemology which occupies the same space as biomedicine, and in drawing upon these spaces they help accomplish and re-accomplish the clinical domain as just that, *clinical*. But at the same time as they hold up the purely clinical space as being at the top of the hierarchy, they incorporate in their gaze a greater scope for the possible influences on a patient's life and health.

As has been shown throughout this book, what is to count as 'medical' trouble is reduced to what can be rendered as clinical. Nurses conduct care in ways which help accomplish this reduction at the same time as they sustain a greater range and scope for interpretation of patients' medical and social futures.

Note

1. It should be noted at this point that not talking with patients was not particularly verified by observation of the nurses at work. Nurses did talk with patients while doing other things for or to them, such as a wash or walking to the toilet, but talk was mainly concerned with chat or focused by nurses on the job in hand. What I think the nurses were aware of was that their talk was not particularly meaningful, what they were not aware of or were not admitting was the extent to which they acted to avoid meaningful talk to control patients' access to them.

Chapter 7

Bedside Care and the Visibility of Nurses' Work

Introduction

The book has examined and made visible how nurses' conduct of care produces ward life in one hospital. The focus has been on the bedside.

At the bedside I watched the comings and goings of nurses, doctors and patients. I also noted the play of inclusions and exclusions, the fluidity of absences and presences, and the conditions of these various exits and entrances.

In this final and concluding chapter I bring these matters together. The chapter begins by summarising the findings of previous chapters. It then goes on to discuss bedside care in relation to the visibility of nurses' work. Finally, it discusses the implications of the study for nursing, for health policy and for the future organisation of the health services.

Nurses: the conductors of care

Chapter 2 illustrated how the multiple agendas that nurses accomplish are made present in their day-to-day lives. First, the hospital has a front: first class, traditional British medicine. In line with this front, nurses are seen to be concerned with appearing as acute medical nurses. At stake is the preservation of a hospital in which acute medicine and nursing is provided, rather than other kinds of care.

Second, the health service as a system under strain from a new managerial agenda is also made obvious. Devices such as the waiting system make demands for shorter lengths of stay and greater efficiency, the other realities nurses are faced with in their day-to-day lives.

The third, more implicit agenda is the call of nursing theory to take all of a person's 'needs' into consideration. Yet nurses more than anyone else are aware of the discrepancy between a professional emphasis on doing what patients say they need and the demands of caring for more than one person in a service situation.

Nurses reconcile these three agendas through distinguishing between different kinds of needs. To do this they relegate some needs as *social* and others as *medical*. Thus, nurses engage in practices which discriminate between patients, denigrating those who are not viewed as medical. To maintain their visibility and preserve their identity, nurses align their work with the technical and heroic work of the clinical domain. In doing so, they constitute social needs and patients with either personal or social problems as 'other'.

Chapter 2 made it clear that there is organising work to do, but it also illustrated the paradox that the appearance of first class medicine depends upon its purity. To keep patients moving through the beds requires particular kinds of organising work, and, as has been shown, the purity of the clinical domain relies on keeping this work backstage.

Chapter 3 reviewed how nurses organise ward life. Processes such as handovers, ward routines, the allocation of work and the placing of patients were examined. Nurses emerge as the *conductors of care*.

Nurses' organisation of the clinical domain depends upon a continuous labour of division. This ongoing labour is present in every aspect of nurses' work, from the placing of patients to the use of routines. Through it nurses differentiate patients, types of work and types of nurses in relation to hierarchies of significance. To fabricate the clinical domain, nurses engage in 'a constituting of classes'. This includes privileging their work with the acutely ill who require frequent observation and much technical care. However, as has been stressed, nurses are not free to decide how ward life should be ordered or care conducted. Rather, they appear to be the conduits through which power effects are made possible.

In particular, nurses make themselves visible as disciplined and knowledgeable. Patients and junior student nurses have no authority – the authority to speak comes with the discipline of the medical gaze. Nurses are thus complicit in the effacement of their other work at the bedside and so their care of patients as sentient beings remains unspoken and invisible. It is relegated to the status of routine.

Nurses also produce ward life in ways that maintain the front of the building, the impression that the acute medical domain is organised on a purely clinical basis. It is not that nurses follow orders. On the contrary, nurses regulate themselves and provide the context in which patients can be viewed as appropriate or inappropriate to the medical domain. To maintain their visibility of doing purposeful and rational work, nurses align themselves with the purity of the clinical domain.

Chapter 4 discussed how the front and backstage work of medicine is distributed between nurses and doctors. The ward round is a spectacle which, like the front entrance of the hospital described in Chapter 2, celebrates and reaffirms British medicine. The ward round maintains the appearance that medicine proceeds on a purely technical and disciplined basis, held apart from the social and the mundane work of organising. But the ward round is also concerned with keeping patients *moving* through the medical domain. Shifting patients from one category to another requires authorisation by the doctors. However, this work involves much more than visualising patients as medical objects; it depends upon nurses' work of contextualising patients' troubles.

Ironically, the nurses' contribution is made to disappear from view. Therefore, even as the spectacle of the ward round rests on the basis of nurses' contextualising work, the ward round itself only makes visible those aspects of nurses' work which are in support of the medical. The other aspects of nursing are subject to an ongoing effacement so that all knowledge and practices which are not easily made technical or clinical are left invisible.

It seems as if it is nurses who are the ones who drive the organisational need for movement and flow, the dirty work of the clinical domain. In reality, nurses are helping doctors to accomplish their agenda – doctors rely on having patients who are good for first class medicine and these are patients who can be seen to recover, patients who are easily processed. This is an agenda that is much more hand in glove with the managerial agenda than is usually recognised. For example, those patients who block the flow are also those who do not fit the medical bill. But in being seen as the ones who do the dirty work of organising, it is the nurses' identities that risk being downgraded. In bearing the brunt of these aspects of hospital work, nurses help maintain the purity of clinical decisions as the doctors' prerogative.

Chapter 5 examined nurses' relationships with patients at the time of their admission to the wards. Nurses' conduct of the admission period initiates patients into the social organisation of the medical domain. Through their encounters with nurses, patients learn how to conduct themselves to maintain their inclusion as good clinical materials. Critically, patients must efface themselves as social beings to be rendered appropriate medical objects. This includes allowing others to authorise their needs.

Patients learn that 'authority', to define what is significant and to legitimate action, lies far from the bedside, not in the nurse–patient relationship. But even more importantly they learn that, in the clinical domain, you only get allocated to the acute class of patient if you allow this effacement to happen. As Foucault (1976) puts it, the performance of clinical medicine depends upon the abstraction of the patient as well as the doctor as a social being. This abstraction requires patient complicity.

Those patients who cannot efface themselves are at risk of being rendered as old and social or, even worse, as vegetable matter, rather than sick. Ironically, in not attempting to promote interpersonal and democratic relations with patients, nurses are helping both themselves and patients to maintain their dignity and their inclusion as proper to the clinical domain. Only this effacement allows their transformation from person to patient (and back again).

Chapter 6 explored nurses' accounts to elaborate how nurses have developed a 'nursing gaze'. Nurses have extended the medical gaze to survey a patient's psychosocial life as well as their progress and behaviour. Nurses *hierarchise* their methods for assessing patients' needs. At the top of the hierarchy is their work of observing patients in relation to medical discourse. At the bottom is their personal knowledge of a patient derived from simply being with them over time. But at the same time as they hierarchise these matters, nurses insist on keeping all potential grounds for viewing patients and understanding their troubles in play. Critically, for nurses, quality of life, assessed by knowing someone over time, must remain possible grounds on which to treat a patient.

Nurses and the bedside

What I found in this study was something very different from what I had expected to find. Instead of the bedside being a site of care, centred by nurses as the touchstone to which understandings, observations and bits of information are continuously referred, nursing assessment is displaced. Instead, the bedside is made up of three social spaces.

The first is constituted by the medical gaze. This gaze constitutes the bedside as a *treatment* space. The person admitted to the bed is denuded of their distinguishing social and personal 'props' and is remade as a patient. 'Patients', as opposed to persons, are composed of networks of artefacts, such as machines, drips, observations and charts. Patients are further extended through forms of writing, such as the nursing profile and the doctor's history and examination. The marks and signs which represent the patient, as he or she is translated into medical discourse, travel back and forth from the bedside through the centres of calculation, at the ward round and the nurses' handover. The signs which are taken to represent the patient are aligned and assigned to a medical category, but they can never remain in a category for too long. Much of nurses' work is concerned with looking for change in patients so that they can be shifted from one category to another.

The second space is composed of the nurses' extended gaze. Through this gaze the bedside is constituted as a space of *movement* and *rehabili-*

tation. Nurses survey the patient for signs that they have the capacity and the will to stop being dependent, to recover, because the medical domain relies on patients being returned to persons. The necessary lack of dependency is, of course, relative and is calculated elsewhere, at the social round, at the nurses' handover and during the ward round. The limits of non-dependence are set relative to the resources available to support the older person at home and to their previous capability, their 'social history'. These matters are continuously assessed by nurses. They survey the patient's relationships, conduct and progress to assess their moral, functional, social, emotional and mental situation.

The nursing process and geriatric assessment have technologised and institutionalised nurses' extended gaze. But, critically, its legitimation has come through the managerial imperative for movement. Through contextualising patients' troubles nurses provide the grounds for shifting patients' identities to pull them through the beds. We have seen this in the case of Mrs Weston (page 67). Sister got Mrs Weston moving by refiguring her, by shifting her out of one medical category (the acutely ill) into another, someone to be mobilised. Mrs Weston re-emerged in Sister's discourse as other than acutely ill. She was refigured as someone very old, an RTA, an orthopaedic problem – someone at risk of prolonged immobility.

Returning for a moment to the opening of the book, we can understand that it is these activities of observation which make nurses' presence at the bedside feasible as purposeful and important work. Their extended gaze incorporates the medical objectives of diagnosis and effective treatment with the managerial objective of getting patients up and moving through the beds. In this way, nurses' work takes its visibility from orders of discourse coming from elsewhere.

The patient is never involved in the legitimation of significance. As detailed in the analysis of Major Stevenson's admission (page 86), legitimation comes from elsewhere, far from the nurse–patient relationship, and discretion lies in other bodies of knowledge. This connects to the third space which has emerged in the study.

The bedside is also a space of *initiation, transformation* and *passage,* for patients as well as junior nurses. Patients read nurses' conduct and pick up how to conduct themselves. Nurses, exercised by the handover, the nursing records and the admission procedure, convey to patients that, as persons, neither of them has any authority. Nurses convey that it is the effacement of patients as socially differentiated beings that helps them to be figured as worthy of medical diagnosis and care. It is the effacement of the social which allows the transformation of persons into appropriate clinical materials.

Nurses are engaged in these multiple ways of making the patient visible as belonging, or not, to the acute medical domain. Critically, belonging should be momentary and a patient should be quickly on the move, returning to person and returning home.

It follows that nurses are engaged in the *distribution* of medicine in two senses. First, nurses' conduct constitutes the bedside as a space which distributes medicine through the parallel lines of sight incorporated in the nurses' extended gaze. Second, nurses' work helps constitute a patient as in need, or not, of specific types of treatment and care. Mrs Marsh, Mrs Adamson and Mrs Weston (pages 53, 59 and 67) were refigured by nurses as no longer in need of *medical* diagnosis, investigation and treatment. In refiguring these people as no longer appropriate to the acute medical domain, the nurses helped to move them along from an admission to a discharge.

In doing this work of distributing medicine, nurses' conduct organises the clinical domain. Their conduct organises the flow and so nurses help pull patients through the beds, to keep them moving. But nurses also organise the boundaries and the closures – they construct and reconstruct the limits of the acute medical domain.

Critically these spaces at the bedside operate together and are mutually supplementary. Each takes its composition and legitimacy from the centres of calculation and discretion which operate at a distance from the patient (at the notes trolley and at the ward handover). We can consider, then, that the nurses are the *conduits* through which these lines of sight travel to and from the patient. Thus, it is no longer possible to think of the bedside as a simple location: the site of nurture and care. Nor is the bedside a site of negotiation, in which nurses can decide with patients what it is that they need. The bedside has been reconfigured as a space of observation, not as a site of involvement, and the nursing station emerges as the centre of calculation.

But nurses are ambivalent toward their conduct of care and comply with processes which hide or downgrade it. This is because nurses' conduct of care is deeply problematic.

The mundane work of nursing

Nurses' conduct is problematic. Critically, the ordering of the clinical domain engages nurses in practices of inclusion and exclusion – in real life nurses cannot align with all of their patients. Nurses' conduct of care as we have seen it therefore does not fit models of nursing because these stress that nurses should base their relations either on a heroic and traditional professional–client model, or on the new professionalism which democratises nurse–patient relations (Salvage, 1992; Davies, 1995; Benner, 1996)[1].

But nurses' work is problematic for other reasons. It is not just that it involves the 'dirty work' of caring for and 're-covering' (Rudge, 1996) the disordered body. In contrast to Lawler's (1991) analysis, acute care nurses increasingly organise the clinical domain so that this work is undertaken by others – 'ordinary' women clean patients' bodies and domestics serve them meals. Nor does simply gendering nurses' organising work explain the complexity. It is not just that nurses' work is, as Davies (1995) stresses, discounted because it is domestic and private – women's work.

Nurses' conduct of care is not constituted by nurses themselves as either caring or clinical work. Indeed, as we have seen in Chapter 2, one staff nurse stated that she considered her organising work as against caring, as somehow against the individualising of nursing care. Nurses' conduct of care has no place in current theoretical categories. As such it remains invisible, it cannot be named. Therefore, nurses' conduct of care is problematic, partly because it is betwixt and between categories, and as such it is potentially polluting (Douglas, 1966).

There is another reason why nurses' conduct is problematic and why it is so difficult to name. Nurses engage in discourses of differentiation and classification. But nurses' systems of distinction are not just based upon clinical processes, those of differential diagnosis. This would be fine if it were so – everyone would agree this is what they are supposed to do. The difficulty is that nurses' systems of distinction draw processes of *social* differentiation into the medical domain. These practices are deeply problematic where the association between positive identity and clinical, rather than social, practices is acted out in almost everything else nurses do. But the insistence on the purity of the clinical domain is itself a perverse act of *social* purity. Thus, in a world dominated by notions deriving from the politics of identity, the fact that nurses survey patients as persons to help support clinical decisions is deeply problematic. It is not that nurses simply act out social prejudices, as earlier sociologists have claimed; there is nothing personal and nurses are not simply reifying good and bad patients. On the contrary, as has been seen, nurses are extremely careful to individualise their distinctions between types of patients. Not all older people, for example, are distinguished as having problems due to their age. Instead, it is nurses' practices of distinction which provide the flexibility necessary for keeping patients on the move.

Nurses' organising work is not just in dramatic opposition to nursing theory, which limits nurses to relations with individual patients and which promotes the democratisation of the nurse–patient relationship. It also risks the purity of the clinical domain. Even though, as we have seen in Chapter 6, nurses technologise their survey of patients' social and emotional lives, these practices associate nurses with those acts of exclusion upon which all organising is based, but which the clinical domain must efface to maintain its purity as 'socially impartial'.

Nurses' work is therefore polluting because it engages nurses in what are made to appear as *non-clinical* practices of differentiation. The problem then is with how 'the clinical' is constructed, as if it is based on non-social practices, and the perpetuation of the *purity* of the clinical domain which effaces all the 'social' work which goes on in medicine. I believe that the need for this purity has been reinforced by the logic of the new management and a particularly narrow definition of rationality and purposefulness, of evidence and efficacy.

The difficulty facing nurses (and some doctors) is how to rewrite what constitutes (good) medicine. This paradox is, I believe, of relevance to the difficulties in both recruiting and retaining nurses. This is considered in the following section.

Any future for nursing?

Nurses have emerged in this book as strong and knowledgeable women doing important work that goes far beyond the stereotypical picture of them. Nurses achieve quality acute care in a context dominated by medical objectives and reinforced by the politics of the waiting list. Quality is defined by the demands of 'management by objectives' and 'first class medicine.'

Critically, in the context of contemporary medical and health policy agendas, not all patients or types of work will do. Work must be visible as purposeful and rational, yet work that has visibility is limited to the attainment of clinical and managerial objectives. Patients who have problems which do not resolve speedily are constituted as 'other'. We have seen how patients like 'bay 4 ladies' are dismissed as 'vegetable matter'; Mrs Marsh, as the 'pea lady', almost literally so.

Under these conditions, the bedside has been transformed. Care at the bedside is becoming less and less visible, more and more social, or 'not-clinical'. The long-term implications of this invisibility are immense. First, nurses are being forced to abandon (to care assistants or to informal carers, Gregor, 1997) the work at the bedside which is the very work which makes nursing distinct from other health professions. Second, to stay visible, nurses are taking on more and more medical tasks and technologising their practices. Both these effects risk excluding the kind of nurses who want to look after and care for people in a traditional way. Nursing is losing its appeal as a woman's profession, its appeal to people who want a vocation, a calling, rather than a job.

For others, traditional nursing has a problematic identity because of the association between nursing and women (see Davies, 1995; Rafferty, 1996). Yet as we have seen, this view was too simplistic. As women, traditional nurses moved between the patient at the bedside and the doctor's ward rounds. As women *in between*, then, nurses were human, if barely visible. But things have changed. The competing demands of professionalising agendas and of health service managers have led to a 'technologising' of nurses. Now nurses are expected to do more than care, or extend the doctors' gaze in their absence. Instead, nurses move between the technologies of nursing accountability and health service managers' demands for greater service efficiency. In this changing picture, nurses re-emerge as moving *in between* the bedside as a site of exclusion and the nurses' station as a centre of calculation. Nurses' relationships with patients have become technologised in new ways – nurses are half-human, half-machine.

Within this new framing any demonstrable gain from traditional care and compassion now seems impossible to prove. Research must move on to study the effects of the new technologies and not dwell on tradition, in case it seems nostalgic. But I will suggest here that there is a relation between why nurses are no longer entering the service as a vocation, and the exclusion of those practices which are demeaned as social rather than health care work. A new labour of division is not only dehumanising the health services, but changing the face of nursing.

Note

1. The following quote from Benner exemplifies:
   'In the context of generous knowledgeable caring practices that are finely tuned by one's own sentient and skilled embodiment, the level of mutual respect and knowledge of the other will allow for more than mere rights and justice. *The language of cost–benefit analysis and other forms of rational calculation* will seem like impoverished 'outside-in-accounts' that miss the human connection and community and particular human concerns in the situation.' (Benner, 1996, p. 253; emphasis added)
   Ideologically, I am completely 'in tune' with Benner's call here, but it demeans nurses' accomplishments in the tough world of contemporary health care.

Endnote

Geertz (1995) tells us how he always felt he arrived at the sites of his ethnography 'after the fact'. He felt that key happenings had always just come to an end, or were being anticipated, so it was as if he always seemed to have 'been there' at the time in between. Later he realises that change is impossible to observe.

In contrast, I think that I was doing my ethnography at a key moment in the history of medicine and health care, in Britain at least. This was a moment when nursing's bid for recognition, in the form of a widespread adoption of the 'nursing process', overlapped with more general changes in the activities and contentments of women seeking to establish their knowledge as knowledge, rather than as traits of a gendered nature. On the one hand, then, I see the nursing process as a material-discursive practice through which nurses exercise (Foucault, 1979) themselves as problem-solvers and decision-makers. On the other hand, doctors, beginning to feel the compelling pressure of accountability in relation to cost and time, are retreating from the bedside of care. It was a moment in which doctors seem to have allowed the inclusion of new practices, such as geriatric and nursing assessment, at the same time as they are aligning themselves with bodies that give a more reliable and positive knowledge than the flesh and blood patient can reveal, namely the machines. It was a moment too in which, despite an absence of any close examination of them at work, nursing and medicine were abandoned as the pinnacles of vocational expertise. A moment in which an even less tried and tested discipline – managerialism – was put in place to change them both and ensure value for money and fitness for purpose.

There are of course many stories around to explain the necessity for all this change. Yet, even today, looking back at the moment in which the destiny of the NHS changed irrevocably, I do not feel these stories to be satisfactory. It is not enough to say that the nature of care is changing because nurses and doctors are having to consider how they care for populations and communities, rather than just for individuals. We have certainly heard how these are available grounds on which practitioners can account for what they see and know as uncaring conduct in relation to the individual. However, it is not enough to explain what we have seen only in terms of competing interests over the distribution of time, space and resources. There is much more at stake, culturally and ethically, particularly over the comprehensiveness of health services and their flexibility to individuality, both of staff and of patients.

I hope this book helps to excavate how medicine is a *distributed* practice, one in which nurses, doctors, patients and many other human and non-human actors participate. Critically, I want to emphasise how the invisibility of the social is being exaggerated and further squeezed by the relentless emphasis on increasing turnover to reduce waiting lists, coupled with an evidence-based movement grounded on a particularly narrow interpretation of proof and rationality.

The participants in this study attempted to accomplish their organisation as a purely medical enterprise, an agenda which involved the traditional success stories of cure, self-care and rehabilitation. These will go on. However, even as participants were failing in these narratives, they also showed themselves to be immensely resourceful at holding in play social and other grounds in order to help shift the identities of patients. This mobility helps justify how (some) older people are appropriate patients for (acute) medical and nursing attention. Of course, illness and disability, particularly in old age, cannot always be talked up to fit in with wider fashions.

In holding the patients at a distance, the doctors and nurses figured and refigured some of them as having identities which were appropriate to a medical domain. But in the older body, pathology is frequently multiple, sometimes chronic, sometimes acute and temporary, so stabilising the body's functions to allow for medical treatment and intervention is risky in an environment which is itself under strain. Remember how, for older people, the usual orders can be reversed – 'she's 88, get her going'. And so out she goes, for it is difficult either to accomplish or trace, and therefore prove, the success of medical practices and interventions in a body in which the variables are so difficult to control and in which illness is never complete until death has overtaken it. Indeed, new pressures are making it even more tempting to find ways to constitute older people as having conditions that make medical treatment futile, a waste of time and money. After all, even as subjects for randomised control trials, older people fail.

Already in the short time since this study was finished, the new management has introduced further pressures on health service practitioners and has made available even more reasons for excluding the many different types of patient from accessing professional nursing care. For example, added to the pressure of increased throughput is an insistence on medicine as a success story of *completed* diagnostic episodes and clinical pathways. This seems to me to be forcing conditions under which even the minimalist care we have seen is in danger. In the situation we are now facing, practitioners will be pressed into reducing treatment even further if they are to meet all the demands upon them.

Looking forward now, is there a possible end to the tyranny of transparency and explicitness? If care resides in the space between the visible and the unsaid, but where there can never be a simple return, what sort of culture would permit the creation of a new space at the bedside? A space where it is permissible to care.

Appendix 1

Theoretical Nursing Assessment: the Construction of a Profession

Nursing assessment is probably one of the most important things nurses do as it includes those practices and processes through which a patient's 'troubles' are translated into needs. And yet there is very little research on nursing assessment as an aspect of nurses' everyday conduct.

Usually, in representations of nursing assessment, its peculiar and unique character appears to lie in how it may take into account any aspect of a patient's life, to understand how his (or her) illness may be impacting, spiritually, physically, functionally, socially or psycho-emotionally. Thus, nursing assessment can be understood to bring 'non-medical' dimensions of health and illness into play within the medical domain. These aspects of the character of nursing assessment are emphasised as even more crucial in circumstances where the effects of illness may be long term, life threatening or simply multiple and complicated, as in the case of the chronically sick, the dying or older people.

However, there is another less explicit aspect to nursing assessment, which is more difficult to represent. Nursing assessment, as written in narratives of caring, *centres* the patient, not just as an object to be observed, informed or consulted, as in discourses of customer care, but as a feeling, experiencing and knowledgeable subject, located in a specific and unique social and material context. It is only where nurses place themselves in relation with, not to, the patient as a situated person that his or her needs can emerge accurately and appropriately.

In representing nursing assessment in this way it is being located in an interpretative paradigm in which understanding, as well as knowledge, is being stressed. But what is also being stressed is that interpretation, and the identification of need, are *interactively* constituted, so that a need is not a given but a matter of interpretation, situated, both socially and materially, between persons and things (like thermometers or ECG machines). However, what is also being drawn upon is the idea that it is the nurse–patient relationship which acts as the central medium through which all understandings of need must 'pass'. I mean that in both senses of the term – orders and discourses located through evidence, or in professional bodies of knowledge such as medical discourse, are of use. However, the understandings or knowledge which they help produce about patients and their troubles must be drawn into and *checked* against this other space, continuously created between nurses and patients at the bedside.

The space at the bedside emerges as symbolic of this interactive relationship between nurses and patients through which all interpretations (which result in the identification of a need) must be passed. It is the bedside which is the space of discretion for nurses in their assessment of patients' needs. This particular siting of care does, however, rely upon nurses aligning themselves with patients rather than with other bodies of knowledge.

However, this said, the processes and practices associated with nursing assessment have to date mainly been represented and researched in terms of abstract educational models of problem-solving and decision-making, or through narrative and retrospective accounts of care which continuously re-centre understanding and judgement in the nurse as professional.

Nursing assessment, conceptualised or 'written' as a stage in the nursing process, is located at the bedside in interaction with the patient and nurse, who are figured as individuals. However, in representations of nursing assessment, the nurse arrives at the bedside informed by 'theory' and carrying documents which, once filled in, will help her to decide what the patient's problems are and what she (or someone else) needs to do about them. The interaction is thus (in theory) structured through the inscriptions on the form, and the skills and routines the nurse has learnt to fill in the forms. The nurse is 'looking' at the patient, questioning them and listening to them, but as a naturalist, 'according to a grid of perceptions' and a code for notation (Foucault, 1991), the validity, veracity and good sense of which are located in understandings composed elsewhere. The bedside is thus refigured as a new space of revelation, structured through the routinised practices of the nurse with her special skills.

Nursing assessment is thus prescribed as a primarily *cognitive* activity which involves information processing and problem identification, or 'diagnostic reasoning' (see Roper *et al.*, 1980, 1981). There are three important effects of locating nursing assessment in the cognitive model. First, the cognitive model implies that patients' needs are givens, matters of fact waiting to be detected or revealed through the appropriate application of the skilled and educated nursing gaze. In this sense, nursing assessment has been written in ways which fall into line with other professional practices that help to identify its practitioners with objectivity and with having special skills and sight, such as the medical examination and history (Foucault, 1976). Second, nursing assessment is conceived of as a 'stage' in the nursing process. As such it is a form of management by objectives. In this way nursing assessment emerges as a managerial technology (see also Walton, 1986) which will help to make nurses more accountable (see Pearson & Vaughn, 1986) and, I would aver, more visible to non-nurses. This accountability is (supposedly) accomplished through making nurses think in terms of the individual patient and their specific problems, for which they must find a rational solution which then becomes the objective which all activity must be aimed at accomplishing. This emphasis on nursing assessment as predictive and as a problem-solving and decision-making activity implies that the fact-finding will move to a second stage: the identification of problems and, importantly, the *closure* of a decision. Care cannot be constituted through a mere response or as discontinuous acts – if care is not reflected upon and is not the result of a decision, it is in some way irrational and, as such, unaccountable. Finally, as a stage in the nursing process, nursing assessment is not being written as continuous but as a set of discrete 'problem-solving' activities, even if these are circuitous. This suggests that nurses can detach the work of patient assessment from their other work, for example, of managing and organising wards, clinics or caseloads.

Writing nursing assessment in this way does not only enrol the symbols of the enlightened thinker to talk up nurses as professionals, but it may also enrol nurses in a particular version of knowledge and power. While displacing the important contributions of nurses to health care, the nursing process, which is aimed at making the rational underpinnings of nurses' practices visible, can also be considered as an always failing technology of control that may, ironically, precisely help to keep nurses' accomplishments hidden.

Emphasising the cognitive aspects of nursing assessment has come in for much criticism as being unrepresentative of nursing reality. Nursing assessment as a stage in the nursing process has been considered mechanistic and instrumental (Hiraki, 1992), and as having a disciplining effect on patients (Bloor & McIntosh, 1990; May, 1991, 1992; Purkis, 1993) and on nurses themselves (Hiraki, 1992; Latimer, 1995). In particular, nursing assessment, as a stage in the nursing process which locates accountability for decisions and care with the individual nurse, can be understood as an (always failing) technology of control (Latimer, 1994, 1995), as just one device through which practice discipline is maintained through a 'regulated autonomy' (Rose & Miller, 1992). As a technology it may help divide nurses from each other to make them easier to rule (Dingwall *et al.*, 1988) and, through forms of inscription, compel nurses to attend to those aspects of patient care which are reducible to a problem (Latimer, 1994). The 'rest' gets forgotten, excluded, remains private, ad hoc, a matter of luck.

The critique of the nursing process which has been most pronounced, however, has come from those writers who stress the embodied and interpretative nature of nursing knowledge. Henderson, for example, reintroduces the notion of the embodied subject:

'...the point has perhaps been made that reducing the nurses' function to an analytical, more or less objective process divorces it from the intuitive, subjective response.' (Henderson, 1981, p. 108)

Crow *et al.* (1995) also stress the importance of understanding nursing assessment as situated practices to suggest that nurses are doing more than simply identifying problems; they are also making evaluations and judgements.

Currently, Benner (Benner, 1984, 1996; Benner & Tanner, 1987; Benner & Wrubel, 1989; Benner *et al.*, 1992) is the main advocate for developing an interpretative or phenomenological theory of nursing expertise, through a focus on skill acquisition, patient assessment and clinical judgement. While Benner (1984) accepts the information-processing, problem-identification model as the conceptual model or framework through which nurses learn how to assess patients, she has argued that the ways in which nurses 'know' what patients need is not simply enhanced by practice and experience, but is actually changed through practising nursing to become expert (Benner *et al.*, 1992).

In Benner's approach there remains an object – the subject patient and their needs – which can come into view through a correct reading and interpretation of signs and symptoms. But what Benner adds is the notion that a proper reading is situated and interpretative, it requires the situated engagement of the subject nurse with the subject patient, as well as with other actors, such as doctors.

Thus, although the ways in which nursing assessment is being con-stituted have shifted in the interpretative approach to include the nurse as embodied subject, there remain difficulties. Nurses' assessments remain firmly located in both dyadic relations and within a paradigm of expertise, where the individualised nurse arrives at a judgement or decision. The nurse as subject embodies (or does not) the prerequisite knowledge, skills *and* values to interact (appropriately or not) with her environment (her patient, the doctor, other nurses) to produce meanings which then lead to a clinical judgement.

The specific ways in which nursing assessment is being constituted in the literature are further reflected in the ways in which it has been researched. Nurses' assessments of patients, or their judgements, have rarely been studied directly in the practice setting, except in relation to specific 'assessment events', such as patient admissions (see Faulkner & Maguire,

1984; Price, 1987) or assessment rounds (Morrison, 1989). Most studies of nurses' assessment practices rely on retrospective accounts (Benner, 1984), or simulated patient cases (Hurst & Dean, 1987; Tanner *et al.*, 1987; Hurst *et al.*, 1991; Thiele *et al.*, 1991). Nursing assessment is constituted as 'clinical' in these ways, and possible relations between nurses' practices and wider organisational and social issues are either only brought into play at the moment where there is a 'problem' with the ways in which nurses assess their patients (see Wells, 1980; Melia, 1981; Faulkner & Maguire, 1984; Faulkner, 1985; Price, 1987; Ward, 1988) or, by being treated as mundane, are deleted altogether. Benner, for example, states that she is setting out to identify 'the knowledge embedded in clinical practice' (1984, p. 1), but that the goal 'was not to describe the typical day or hour but rather the highlights, the *growing edges* of clinical knowledge' (p. xxi).

Benner's displacement of the everyday to focus on what is a highlight or extraordinary constitutes a reification of nursing knowledge. Specifically, the complex, heterogeneous and daily world of nursing is treated merely as a background to nurses' thinking, and the ways in which they assess people as patients with needs. This detachment can be understood as helping to constitute the narrative of clinical nursing practice, as a domain which is separate from the everyday, mundane and polluting work of managing or organising.

> 'In the context of generous, knowledgeable, caring practices that are finely tuned by one's own sentient and skilled embodiment, the level of mutual respect and knowledge of the other will allow for more than mere rights and justice. The language of cost–benefit analysis and other forms of rational calculation will seem like impoverished "outside-in-accounts" that miss the human connection and community and particular human concerns in the situation.' (Benner, 1996, p. 253)

This insistence on the purity and heroism of nurses' clinical practice which transcends the mundane world of the everyday (which, astonishingly, even includes matters of rights and justice, as well as resources and funding!) has its advantages. The nurse is positioned as an individual who determines her own destiny. As such she is represented as having a choice between aligning herself with the patient, as other, in a spiritual and unworldly communion (notice the almost religious overtones), or getting caught up in instrumentalism and rational calculation, the world of organisation, and politics and, it has to be said, power. But this way of writing nursing may not just constitute a 'methodological romanticism' (Silverman, 1989). It may also backfire, as nurses remain stranded, isolated as mere individuals who are strategically impoverished in the discourses of organisation and policy.

There are risks in representing or *writing* nurses in these ways. First, there is a risk that nurses are given the task of the heroes who must disembed themselves from the complex and heterogeneous organisations and societies in which they work (see Lawler, 1991), so that their actions will be misunderstood as failing to live up to a heroic and pure model of practice. Under these circumstances, trained to believe in the myth of unadulterated and unmediated nurse–patient relationships, nurses in practice must somehow make sense of a situation which simply does not live up to the theory and find ways to defend themselves against feelings of guilt and demoralisation (Lyth, 1960). Second, there is a risk that much of the important assessing and organising work nurses do is simply devalued. The study on which this book is based developed an approach to reconsider how nurses assess patients for care which takes into account how nurses work in complex environments (increasingly) concerned with 'delivering a service', as well as providing individual care.

Appendix 2
Older People and Acute Medicine

The setting, a UK teaching hospital, exemplifies a system under 'strain' (Giddens, 1984). During the 1980s and early 1990s pressure in the 'acute sector' of the health services came from a number of different directions.

First, a managerialist climate penetrated the health service which led to an 'examination' of the health service and the use of resources (Walton, 1986; Strong & Robinson, 1990; Broadbent *et al.*, 1991; Davies, 1995). Under this examination there was increasing pressure to justify the use of acute sector beds as the most expensive health service commodity. An effect of this has been the emphasis on the need to reduce waiting lists, partly by increasing throughput. Throughput (now referred to as 'completed consultant episodes') has emerged as a measure of efficiency and effectiveness. Further, practitioners across the board were pressed to demonstrate how their practices differed from those who were less expensive to employ. Critically, practitioners have been increasingly under pressure to demonstrate the gain to be had from their activities. The nursing process is just one example of a technology introduced into the acute sector that is aimed at managing practice by objectives (Walton, 1986), but which simultaneously demonstrates the efficacy of practice through making the outcomes of interventions and care visible.

Second, strain arises from the tension created between the perceived purpose of the institution in question – the provision of 'first class medicine' with maximum technology for a class of patient termed the 'acutely ill' – and the limited resources available. Specifically, there has been pressure from the presence of older people in the acute sector. This becomes a problem where there is pressure to increase turnover and demonstrate outcomes in the light of various claims: claims about an increasing older population; claims that older people get ill and are disabled more often than younger people; claims that older people take longer to get out of hospital than younger patients; and, finally, claims that older people require not just medical, or technological, but more so-called 'rehabilitative' and 'socially aware' care. This situation has given rise to the notion of 'bed blocking' and of older people as potential 'bed blockers' (McArdle *et al.*, 1975; Rubin & Davies, 1975; Seymour &

Pringle, 1982; Donaldson, 1983; Barker *et al.*, 1985; Coid & Crome, 1986).

In these ways 'older people' becomes a specifically distinct category of person which is linked negatively with time, given the pressure to increase throughput. Older people are constituted in many different ways but an aspect of these identities is that they can pose a possible impediment to the effective and efficient management of the acute sector, where this is measured by shorter lengths of stay and increased throughput. Statistically, older people acted on 'as a block' (Goffman, 1978) can be identified as increasing the risk of failures over throughput. The care of 'old persons' becomes a target to be managed.

Managers need to know what is different about older people and the care they require. These distinctions relate to explanations for why the length of hospital stay increases with advancing age. The literature reviewed suggested three groups of factors that influence the length of stay of older patients in acute wards. In summary, these are:

(1) Complicated responses to and types of illness: multiple pathology, chronic and disabling diseases, greater vulnerability to stress. These legitimate the problem of older people as falling within a medical terrain.
(2) Inadequate management of patient care. This indicates how there needs to be expertise of a different kind to develop efficient approaches to the care of older people. The emphasis is on comprehensive assessment and the interrelationship between medical issues and the non-medical, that is home life and support, as well as mental, functional and emotional issues which can affect the recovery and rehabilitation of older people.
(3) 'Misplacing' of the old as a result of insufficient or misused alternative care arrangements and resources.

The first group of factors relate to claims that physical and mental aspects of being old may inhibit recovery. In addition to an increased likelihood of multiple health problems, disease in old age is claimed as frequently disabling and increasingly chronic in nature (Hamdy, 1984). Further, older people, it is claimed, have less reserve capacity with which to cope with physical and mental stress (Brocklehurst, 1978, 1982; Jolley, 1987; MacLennan, 1987). This can result in a greater vulnerability to the disabling effects of acute episodes of illness, hospital admission and prolonged inactivity (Brocklehurst, 1978; Gillick *et al.*, 1982; Seymour & Pringle, 1982; Miller, 1984; Hulter Asberg, 1986). In this way the claims relate to producing classifications based upon physiological, that is 'natural', and acceptable, medical criteria for older people's longer recovery times. At the same time these distinctions place older people as potentially requiring different facilities from those represented by acute medicine. This opens a gap: that older people are not like acutely ill patients, they are different.

The second group of factors indicate that deficits in the medical and nursing 'management' of the care of older people in the acute sectors may also contribute to prolonged hospital stays (Rubin & Davies, 1975; Burley *et al.*, 1979; King's Fund, 1982; Barker *et al.*, 1985). Deficits arise from the fact that the assessment of need and organisation of care are not developed from a real understanding of the potential care requirements of acutely ill older people. These studies indicate that caring for older people requires additional expertise to that developed traditionally in the acute ward environment. Older people require so-called comprehensive assessment, with an emphasis on rehabilitation, early discharge planning and strong multi-disciplinary and community liaison.

The third set of factors relate to the availability of alternative care arrangements. Inappropriate or insufficient facilities and support both inside and outside the hospital may result in inappropriate admission to hospital (Currie *et al.*, 1979) and inhibit discharge arrangements (Bouchier & Williamson, 1982; Victor & Vetter, 1984, 1985). Within the hospital environment, in addition to medical and nursing care, resources which are important to the care of older people include remedial therapies, medical social work, and the provision of appropriate equipment (Bouchier & Williamson, 1982; King's Fund, 1982). Outside the acute hospital unit there is the question of the availability of alternative suitable accommodation in the geriatric, psychogeriatric, terminal care or social service sectors. There is also the question of the availability of community support. This can be formal – in relation to community nursing, day care, personal social services and voluntary organisations – or informal – family, neighbours and friends. The problem here is that these 'facilities', first, may not be available and, second, may not be utilised adequately even if they are (Rubin & Davies, 1975; Burley *et al.*, 1979).

Problematising and focusing on how to 'manage' the care of older patients in the acute sector can be seen, then, to revolve not simply around the medical condition of the patient but also around time and cost. It also helps to configure the bed, and the bedside, as a resource which has to be distributed, but effectively and appropriately.

Thus, comprehensive assessment had become as crucial a factor as diagnosis in the efficient and effective management of older people in acute care contexts. This then means that there is another very good reason for the emergence of nursing assessment in an acute medical ward – to facilitate methods of dealing with the problem of older people. Nursing assessment helps focus nurses' attention on a patient's functional and social situation and so it is a complementary tool to geriatric assessment.

The questions that were facing managers and staff at the time of the study were how to prevent older people from being admitted unnecessarily to an acute hospital, and how to speed up the process of getting older people through the hospital and out the other side, at the same time as ensuring that they were properly and safely provided for. I believe that one of the reasons I was so readily funded and accepted into the hospital was because people were hoping that my research on the assessment of older people in an acute medical unit might contribute to solutions to the problem of bed blocking.

Appendix 3
Methods and Methodology

The aim of this book is to help rethink the ways in which health care is being practised, in Britain at least. While it is usually doctors who are considered the key figures in health care, and who are the focus of much medical sociology and health care policy, I believe this is problematic because it may help to reproduce a particular and unitary version of medical practice and medical knowledge as solely the domain of doctors, rather than as distributed. I have centralised nurses, partly to help relocate medical practices as precisely distributed, and because, in hospital at least, it is the relationships between nurses and patients at the bedside which are traditionally figured as the site of caring practices. However, as can be seen in the book, doctors' practices have dramatic effects on the figuring of patients' and nurses' identities.

The methodological approach was chosen to ensure a meticulous collection of material. This involved two important strategies. The first was the structuring of the collection of research material to enable different views to be cross-checked, so that what occurred at the bedside could be verified against records of events in documents, accounts and stories recorded on ward rounds and at nursing handovers. In this way, I travelled with representations of patients across different locations and noted their transformations. Second, following Strathern (1991), during the analysis and transcription of the study I have continually held up the practices and relationships which I found against different discourses, both within the writing on nursing and medicine and outside, in the world of health policy and social theory.

To shift understandings of how health care is practised, I have located the range and extent of nurses' conduct within a number of theoretical frameworks about conduct more generally.

First, we look at nurses' work in the context of social relationships. Nurses work alongside others, for example, doctors, managers and cleaners, as well as other nurses and patients. Nurses do not solely belong to a profession, or to Benner's 'community' of patients and nurses (Benner, 1996). Rather, they belong to wards, hospitals or community clinics and general practices. Further, belonging is not necessarily ever finally established – membership, whether it be of an organisation or a profession, can be understood as being performed continuously (Munro, 1996; Strathern, 1995).

Nurses' practices can be understood, then, as not simply functional or instrumental, moral or spiritual, but also as expressive of identity. To belong, nurses perform in ways which help to make them visible, as 'nurses', 'employees', 'professionals', 'colleagues' or 'good'. In other words, nurses carry out 'identity-work' in multiple domains.

Second, the things that constitute the marks which will pass for each of these (good, nurse, employee, colleague, for example) are not simply written through nursing discourse, or dyadic relations and inter-subjectivities between nurses (their embodied skills, knowledge, values and understandings) and their patients. Rather, there is a surveillance dimension to understanding how nurses practise, where their conduct is itself judged. They must indeed judge themselves against criteria or objectives which are not necessarily homogeneous or dictated by pro-fessional issues (see Bruni, 1995; Davies, 1995; Purkis, 1996; Rudge, 1996). Purkis' (1993) study raises the question of why community nurses do not visit families at home. There is the implication that the nurses do not leave the clinic because home visits are difficult for others to see as work, and if they are not visibly working colleagues and managers may think that the nurses are skiving.

Nurses are, therefore, in a position where their actions have to make sense to others. So, if they are to 'get along' and fit in, they must practise in ways which are open to interpretation. Nurses can accomplish this through using materials which make what they are doing seem self-evident (Goffman, 1958), or through giving accounts (Garfinkel, 1967; Gilbert & Mulkay, 1983) which help make what they are doing appear rational, moral and legitimate (Garfinkel, 1967; Giddens, 1984; Silverman, 1993). To make their practices manifestly sensible to others, nurses, like other social actors, are therefore compelled to make use of narratives, dis-courses, and other materials and devices which are culturally and socially available (Strathern, 1992; Mueller, 1995).

Lastly, patients are usually encountered by nurses not as individuals but as one among others, part of a group or caseload of people with a variety of conditions and situations. Nurses, therefore, have a primary role in not just caring in some simplistic sense for 'a patient', but also in organising patients and the workplace to be able to meet many different people's requirements. Importantly, nurses are faced with ensuring that staff and other non-human resources are available and properly deployed. They are involved, in a pragmatic way, in a distribution of resources. Critically, this means that nurses assess one patient's requirements in relation to others'. However, while nurses appear to be doing assessment as individuals, this does not suggest that they have the autonomy to decide which activity or patient should be privileged over others. Rather, the very circulation of power can be seen in relation to how these matters are ranked and decided (Latimer, 1997).

In summary, the methodological approach taken in the study focused on the distinctions which nurses and other professional carers put into play to figure the identities of people as patients with needs. One could consider these distinctions as 'givens', as matters of expert interpretation simply requiring the objective, experienced and informed gaze of the good nurse, doctor, and social worker, the multi-disciplinary team favoured by geriatricians and others concerned with the health and welfare of older people. However, I have taken a different perspective. Along with other sociological and anthropological studies of medical practices (Buckholdt & Gubrium, 1979; Silverman, 1987; Berg, 1992; Becker & Kaufman, 1995) the position taken is that there is a great deal at stake in how health professionals make their distinctions and categorise people as patients for treatment and care. From this point of view, professionals are considered as members of societies, organisations and institutions, but membership is not simply conferred, it has to be worked at, or 'performed'.

Another common view of encounters and interactions is to limit interpretation of what occurs to matters of individual interest. Here, within encounters 'each person adopts a number of positions in which he or she expresses a sense of self, attempts to exert control over others, attempts to construct meaning' (Ritter, cited in Tilley, 1995, p. vii).

Self is something fixed, and the moves people make involve *individuals*. Following an ethnomethodological tradition, encounters between persons can be viewed differently. They are occasioned or situated (Silverman, 1993). Participants do not have selves, which they can or cannot present and they perform within institutional and cultural orders. Critically, such performances help reproduce institutional and cultural orders. Thus, individuals are subjects but their subjectivities are not taken to be the products of individual choice, motivation, prejudice, ignorance or intention. Instead they are 'constituted in specific institutional and discursive practices' (Silverman, 1987, p. 134).

Participants are not performing 'self' as individual (although it may be very important to give the appearance that this is what is being done). Instead 'self' is seen as constituted through participation as a member. Through their everyday conduct each participant performs their membership. In other words, the activities of nurses and doctors, especially those activities concerned with diagnosing and treating patients, can be considered more as a *function* of the organisation or the institution in which they work. Such activities can be construed as helping a performance of self as member and, through this, as helping to produce and reproduce that organisation (Bittner, 1973), society *and* a moral order (cf. Garfinkel, 1967; Silverman, 1993).

For performance to be persuasive of membership, physical activities alone will rarely do. Members' accounts must make what participants do visible as rational or as having rationale. That is, only some accounts will do. What 'counts' is itself situated. Getting to know what will serve as an account is all part of 'doing' (Garfinkel, 1967) nurse, doctor or, for that matter, patient.

Fieldwork and analysis

The study examined how the identities of people as patients with needs are constituted through the practices of nurses and other participants. An ethnographic approach was, therefore, the method of choice, as it allows examination of the specific discursive and institutional practices through which identities are constituted (Silverman, 1987). While participant observation 'at the bedside' was one obvious method for studying the conduct of care, in order to understand the meaning of conduct at the bedside and why patients were cared for (or not), observation of both organisational structures and processes, and of all possible processes through which patients are being 'identified and named' (Garfinkel & Sacks, 1986), was included in the ethnography.

The focus of the study was the assessment and care of twenty people over the age of seventy-five years admitted as 'acute medical emergencies'. The study took place in an acute medical unit in a prestigious British National Health Service teaching hospital and extended over an eight-month period. The unit consisted of one male and one female ward (Wards 1 and 2). Fieldwork included observations of skill mix, availability and use of resources, routines, guidelines, care protocols, admission policies, reporting mechanisms, transcription of all nursing and medical in-patient documentation, and participant observation of the following:

- The admission of the twenty patients from Accident and Emergency Department (A&E) and for subsequent two hour periods at regular intervals during their stay.
- 'Nursing handovers' (or change of shift reports) before and after each period of observation.
- Doctors' ward rounds and the 'social' round or 'geriatric ward round' (a form of multi-disciplinary case conference focusing on people aged sixty-five and over).
- Home assessment visits where these were arranged by the occupational therapist.

In addition to participant observation, and the many occasions during which I talked with patients and their families, I also interviewed each patient at the end of their hospital stay (using a tape recorder). This interview was aimed at exploring their versions of their lives, their troubles and of events in hospital. With this material I could then compare and contrast the ways in which they presented and understood their troubles and experiences in their interviews with the ways they conducted themselves in their relationships with practitioners, and with the ways in which practitioners represented the patients. Towards the end of fieldwork I also interviewed all the qualified nurses in order to extend material relating to the ways in which they underpinned and justified their practices. Analysis of these accounts as 'moral tales' helped make visible the multiple authorities and orders to which the nurses were working, and which prefigured the ways in which they conducted themselves.

All field material was constructed into a 'text' (Silverman, 1993) which was analysed using a constant comparative method (see Baruch, 1981, cited in Silverman, 1993), which drew on aspects of anthropological (Marcus & Fisher, 1986; Strathern, 1991, 1992, 1993, 1995) discourse (Silverman, 1987, 1993; Deetz, 1992; Fairclough, 1992) and conversation analysis (Silverman, 1993). Analysis of field material as a text allowed me to trace the ways in which different patients' identities were being configured, both over time and across interactions, in different registers (written, verbal, electrocardiographic, thermometric, radiographic), in different locations, and by different assemblages of people and things.

Appendix 4
The Nursing Records

Nursing process

A version of the nursing process had been introduced by nursing administration several years before the current research took place[1]. According to one senior nurse it had been introduced because it was 'fashionable'. She said there had been very little 'training' for staff as to how to use it. Prior to its introduction, she told me, nurses collected a minimal amount of data for records. She said that nurses nursed patients according to their diagnosis and to ensure their 'comfort'.

The nursing process used by nurses in this study consisted of forms of documentation called the 'nursing record' (Appendix 7) and had five parts:

- Patient profile
- Care plan
- Columns for operations, investigations and special procedures
- Progress notes
- Discharge checklist[2].

Records for each patient were kept in a sectioned metal folder at the nurses' station, which the nurses referred to as the 'Kardex'. These records, along with the A&E admission slip, formed the basis of the nurses' handovers.

The different aspects of the records were completed at various times: the assessment was completed soon after the patients' admission; the care plan, if compiled, was completed the same day as the admission or, more often, the following day; the progress record was ongoing and filled in at the end of each shift. While nurses were supposed to sign each entry, they did not always sign the care plan or the assessment record, but they did sign the progress notes. The different aspects of the nursing record are now examined in detail.

Patients were 'assessed' on their admission to the wards. An admission procedure was kept in the procedure manual (see Appendix 6) for each ward, but this did not particularly detail how the assessment process was to be operationalised.

There were two parts to the assessment 'instrument' – the nursing 'profile' and the 'care plan'. The patient profile constituted the 'assessment tool' and it had five parts:

- Reason for admission, medical diagnosis, relevant medical history
- Medication
- Demographic information, including religion and next of kin
- Physical assessment
- Social/psychological assessment.

The categories on the profile were organised according to a varied but essentially normative–functionalist view of what nurses 'need' to know about patients. The categories relating to the nurses' assessment of the patients' current and past health status (such as reason for admission, medical diagnosis, relevant medical history and current medications) were grouped together. This had the effect of making 'health', or the absence of it, correlate with what had been treated, with what had been medicalised. Through inscriptions on the form health was implicated as 'medical', that is, it was 'thinkable' as medical. This was a form of signification which legitimated a particular focus for nurses' attention.

The demographic categories pertain to the bureaucratic view of the patient (name and address, date of birth, next of kin, personal belongings, GP). However, according to models of nursing assessment, this information can also contribute to nurses' understandings of a patient's 'social' context. Categories relating to the physical assessment of the patient adhere to a traditional systems view of the patient – 'bowel', 'bladder', 'skin condition', 'diet', 'respiratory' and 'cardiac function', 'allergies'. However, there were also categories relating to the functionalist view – 'sleep', 'mobility', 'hygiene', 'ability to communicate', 'sight/hearing'. As can be seen from the admission procedure manual, nurses were not expected to examine patients physically, except in relation to what were called their vital signs (blood pressure, pulse, temperature and respiration). Nurses in the study were not seen to do a formal physical examination of patients.

Finally, there were categories designed to give a so-called psychological/social view of the patient – 'social activities', 'occupation', 'emotional status', 'family support', 'health services', 'social and voluntary services'.

While it did not adhere to an activities of living model of patient assessment, the instrument was designed to extend nurses' view of the patient. As well as medical diagnosis and history the tool focused nurses' attention on functional, emotional, social and psychological aspects of patients.

From this extended view of the patient, the nurse was supposed to proceed to a plan of care. In the care plan the nurse identified a patient's 'existing or potential problems', and 'long/short-term aims', designed 'planned nursing action' and projected when each intervention could be evaluated. The assessment procedure was underpinned by a problem-solving, decision-making cognitive model. That is:

data collection → problem identification → plan of action → action → evaluation → reassessment

This model was aimed at stabilising practice by making it more pre-dictable, as well as making it more economical by focusing on an indivi-dual patient's actual needs. But let us take a closer look at how the nurses actually used these tools.

Profiling patients

Nurses completed the profile in a mixture of descriptive and evaluative terms. For example, here is an extract from the profile of Miss Hepburn:

Communication: becoming confused
Mobility: okay indoors
Bowel: eats lots of fruit, regular
Hygiene: wash down at sink
Skin: dry

Some categories were not completed in descriptive terms, but simply recorded the result of the nurses' assessment to indicate that there was 'no problem'. For example, here is an extract from the profile of Mr Donald:

Bladder: No problem
Allergies: None known
Sight/hearing: No problems

Some categories were not completed and were left blank. These usually remained blank.

It is worth noting at this point that the nurses on both wards sometimes created a separate category on the assessment form of elderly patients. This they entitled 'Social History'. Under this category the nurses detailed aspects of a person's life, such as who they lived with, the type of accommodation they lived in (such as whether they had stairs at home), and more general comments about how they were, for example 'confused' or 'upset'. These matters all contributed to the assessment of older patients. As we have already seen in the discussion of Jessie in Chapter 2, nurses took these matters to indicate the degree to which the patient had become *older*, in terms of dependency and reduced mental capacity. Knowing about these aspects of patients helped support nurses' broader categorising of patients, such as medical or social. These features of a patient's life did not just help nurses to assess a patient's needs at the time (i.e. in relation to the help they needed to improve their mobility). Rather, the facts about patients elicited by the patient profile helped to provide a context – they extended the medical gaze to incorporate a survey of the patient as a kind of person, a social being who had (or did not have) particular kinds of resources and support. Importantly, the nursing process, like geriatric assessment, brought the social into the medical domain.

Care planning

It became clear shortly after commencing fieldwork that the nurses in Ward 1 did not often use care plans. A patient's 'problems' were very rarely made explicit in the nursing records. Ward 2 had a greater commitment to making care plans and reviewing the ways in which the nursing process was working to improve nursing care. This commitment was focused around improving the ways in which the nursing documents were completed and helping students understand how to complete and compile them. The clinical teacher had a high profile on this ward and, with Sister's encouragement, began to involve student nurses in discussion about their admissions of patients and about the construction of care plans which led on from those admissions. Because of this anomaly I 'counted' how many patients had care plans. This is detailed below.

	Yes	No	?
W1	18	46	7
W2	73	20	4

Of the 18 patients who had care plans in Ward 1, seven of these had been transferred with the patient from other wards such as CCU or the renal unit. Of the 20 patients included in the main study two women and eight men had care plans, while eight woman and two men did not have care plans.

Where care plans were compiled they were not usually written by the student nurse who admitted the patient but by the nurse-in-charge, unless the admitting nurse was a senior student nurse, was working with the clinical teacher or was herself a qualified nurse. Where there were care plans these were typically written around problems of a physical nature and, sometimes but not always, related to issues uncovered in the assessment profile. Often the care plans were directed at the nurses' assessment of patients' 'signs' and 'symptoms'. Typically patients' feelings were not included in the care plan.

Care plans were either directed at instituting a change (such as in a patients' condition or in their behaviour), at preventing a change, or at monitoring for change. There is an example of a care plan written by a staff nurse on Ward 2 for Mr Donald in Appendix 8.

As can be seen the care plan outlined assessment of the patient's 'problems', indicated projected outcomes or aims, and gave instructions as to the ways in which these were to be achieved in relation to nurses' and patients' activities. Some of these were to be carried out by the nurse as she assessed the patient on an on-going basis. For example, Appendix 8 shows that the nurses were to maintain Mr Donald's hygiene in relation to (her assessment of) his ability.

Typically, where there was a care plan this was rarely updated. They remained the same throughout a patient's stay and only addressed issues concerned with a patient's immediate 'problems' identified on admission or shortly after it. However, in Ward 1, care plans were infrequently used (only two of the patients in the main study had care plans). I suggest that the absence of care plans or the rather inept way in which they were used is significant.

First, not being too categorical about a patient's problems allows for much greater fluidity in the connections that can be made about *what* category a patient fits and about *how* their needs can be defined (for example, as social or medical). It is this fluidity which can provide the grounds for keeping someone moving though the beds.

Second, where care plans were used they helped to flag up what was significant and accountable. Most problems focused on the physical or medical aspects of patients' troubles, thus reflecting the priorities and concerns of the acute medical domain.

The nurses' use of the progress notes is discussed in the next section.

Progress reports

The nursing progress report was written at the end of each shift. At the end of the early shift the nurses wrote their own records about the patients for whom they were responsible, but at the end of other shifts the nurse-in-charge wrote the report. The early and night report was written daily for all patients but the late report was only written for patients where there was some 'change'. The nurses took their writing very seriously and spent considerable time on the reports. The less experienced nurses often looked back to what had been written before to know how to format their own report, or discussed it with each other or asked a more senior nurse. In this way the method for writing reports was circulated and aspects of patients were reiterated.

The progress record was supposed to be structured alongside the care plan. The problem number in the care plan was used to indicate the area of nursing being reported upon in relation to the nursing action taken and the patients' progress and nurses' evaluation. An extract from Mr Donald's progress report is included in Appendix 8. It can be seen from this progress report that the nurses wrote it in relation to the problem and actions outlined in the care plan (denoted by the number at the left hand side of the page).

In Ward 1 where care plans were rarely used there were no explicitly identified problems. The nurses in their progress notes stated the action undertaken (such as 'bathed in big bath') or the observation undertaken (four hourly blood pressure). Sometimes they also qualified an action (such as 'managed well with little help') or their interpretations of the activity or observation in relation to the patient's condition or their overall progress. However, while there was no record of a specific, that is, 'identified' problem, problems emerged through the report and particular activities were connected to them. Although there was no particular statement of intent (aim or objective) in the record, the intent was implicit. Figure 1 is an extract from the progress report of Miss Hepburn.

Date	Prob number	Nursing action taken	Progress/evaluation
2/1		Washed at sink in bathroom	Managed well, no assistance required. Still slightly confused.
3/1		Mobilised to toilet overnight. Big bath given. Had dressing practice with O.T.	Mobilising well round the ward and socialising with fellow patients, very cheerful and friendly. Eating small amounts

Figure 1

Miss Hepburn's behaviour was recorded in relation to observations of her mood. While it was unusual for the records to refer to non-physical or medical aspects of patients, it was legitimated in this particular case because the patient was being observed in relation to her 'confusion'. The nurses were well aware that this might have been inhibiting her progress to a new category, that of someone who was ready for discharge.

The focus of the nurses' record in figure 1 pivots around Miss Hepburn's mobility, her 'confusion' and her level of independence. Although there was no care plan in which these matters were overtly stated as significant problems, the nurses were able to pick up and relay that these were the issues which were of central nursing interest. In their talk about Miss Hepburn it became clear that they were concerned that she was what they call 'borderline'; they constantly observed her mobility, mental state and ability to self-care to question her ability to continue to self-care at home.

Notes

1. Tierney (1984) described the nursing process as a 'method', the purpose of which is 'a systematic approach to the provision of individualised nursing care' (p. 835). I have discussed how the nursing process can be considered a technology designed to make nurses' activities more visible at the same time as it makes nurses more accountable elsewhere (Latimer, 1995).
2. The section in the records for 'operations, investigations and special procedures' is used by nurses to indicate any specific observation or collection of specimens and whether these have been collected or completed. The discharge checklist was not used in either ward.

Appendix 5
Ward Routines

Ward life

Nurses organise the delivery of many of the wards' facilities to patients through ward routines.

The early nurses' day begins at 7.30 am, 'giving out' (they do not use the word 'serving') breakfasts, sitting some patients up, making beds, putting out the wash trollies and the linen trollies and 'skips' for the dirty linen. The nurses divide themselves into pairs for these activities – two sitting patients up and two giving out breakfasts.

Patients are either sat up in bed and their bedtable moved into position or sat up in an armchair by their bed for meals; there is no 'dining area' on either ward. The nurses bring chairs and tables from the dayroom where they are stored at night. Nurses ask patients what they would like for breakfast as they go round or give them food provided by the diet kitchen.

In Ward 1 the nurse-in-charge takes the night report at 7.30. 'Handovers' or reports usually take place at the nurses' station. If there is another qualified nurse on duty, she does the morning drug round. In Ward 2 they are experimenting with having all qualified nurses *and* senior student nurses attend the night report. The senior student nurses then either have no further handover or are given brief instructions as to their patients' care.

When a qualified nurse is on her own then she takes the night staff's handover, the drug round and the handover to the early shift. Because of the way in which the off-duty devolves, the qualified nurses most likely to be on their own in the morning are the most junior staff nurses. If the ward is 'short of staff' in the view of whoever is in charge for the shift, then the medication round is done by a qualified nurse on her own with no checker. On Ward 2, two of the staff nurses liked the nurse responsible for the patient whose drugs they are administering to be checker. They would use this time to handover the patient to the nurse as they went round their bay.

After breakfasts are 'given out', some nurses help patients to eat while others start to make beds until the early shift nursing handover. In Ward 1 all the nurses sat down for this handover. In Ward 2 the qualified nurses hand over patients specific to the nurses to whom they had been allocated. During the rest of the morning patients are washed and some dressed. There is another drug round before lunch, which takes place at midday. The nurses give out the lunches and the nurse-in-charge serves them from a dinner wagon standing at the head of or in the middle of the main ward.

The morning is spent mainly on washes, shaves, teeth cleaning, getting patients up and changed, toileting, bed-making, observations and tidying up. Observations of temperature, pulse and blood pressure are routinised for most patients and done at set times: 10 am, 2 pm, 6 pm, 10 pm, 2 am, etc.

Some patients also go for investigations during the morning. There may be special preparations for these investigations which the nurses undertake before the investigation is due. There are also doctors' ward rounds in the morning. After lunches, there is a toileting time and then a rest time until visiting time at 3 pm. Then the early staff write up their nursing reports, going off duty at 3.45.

The late staff come on at 1 pm. The early charge nurse hands over to them at the nurses' station. After this report they take over from the early staff in toileting and getting patients back to bed while the early staff go to lunch. The nurses are not officially told to hand over their patients at this point to the nurses taking over, although sometimes the student nurses were heard to have a quick word with each other to indicate where they had got to.

The nurses (both early and late) then do the 2 pm observations. Some dressings are scheduled for the afternoon. This might also be a time for teaching or for talking to the long-term patients. Teas are given out between 2.30 and 3 pm. The nurses sit patients up again for this and do pressure area care, ready for visiting time. The late nurses go for their break at 3 pm. On their return they might get more patients up, walk patients and do any special nursing procedures. There is another drug round at 5 pm, and the nurses sit patients up, do toileting and pressure areas ready for supper and do the 6 pm observations at about this time. Once again they often split into pairs. Supper is at about 5.30. Evening visiting is between 6 and 7.30. During this time the nurses take their own supper breaks and start to get some of the long-term patients, who have less frequent visitors, ready for bed. After visiting, the nurses get the rest of the patients ready for bed. The charge nurse writes up the nursing records, handing over to the night staff at 8.45 when they come on duty. The late shift go off duty at 9 pm.

The division of labour

The nurses' day is divided into shifts – early, late and night shifts. There is some overlap between shifts to allow for nursing handovers and breaks.

The nurses are divided into three groups – qualified nurses, student nurses and auxiliary nurses.

The work undertaken by each group varies considerably: what evolves is that there are in effect two types of nurse, the supervisors and the supervised. The supervisors talk about patients, 'make decisions' and give instructions. This group consists of the qualified nurses. The second group are the supervised. This group consists of the student nurses and the auxiliary nurses up to a certain point. The lines are not completely fixed: for example, a junior staff nurse might still require some supervision while a nursing auxiliary or a senior student might be left to more or less 'get on with it'.

Supervisors also participate in the bedside care and the ward routines, such as washes, bed-making or meal-giving. This is an important part of the culture of the setting: qualified nurses are all involved in the delivery of care. They explained that when they are 'in charge' this is a necessity – they stated that with the numbers allocated, they cannot remain supernumerary.

However, some of them also claimed that it is only through being with the patients that they really got to know them. Further, in doing the bedside nursing the qualified nurses, including the Sisters, are carrying on a tradition, acting out a discourse – that nursing is about doing practical jobs, nursing patients. This is egalitarian in a sense, that even the most senior ward-based nurses get involved in the basic care and the 'dirt', and it reinforces the conception that real work in nursing is still rooted in bedside care. The nurses still legitimate themselves through being seen to do nursing practically.

However, in practice, being in charge acts as a constraint on a nurse's relationship with patients. The qualified nurses in charge are always very busy so when they care for patients it is in a rushed and hurried way. They are always being pulled back by matters of organisation. The telephone, other nurses or doctors continuously interrupt their work at the bedside.

The supervisors tell the supervised what they should do in respect of individual patients at handovers and supervise them throughout the shift, sometimes letting them know about changes in care. The supervised contribute to the assessment of patients, and to the making and giving of instructions about care in restricted ways. They carry out the work and give informal verbal reports or formal written reports of aspects of what they have done or what they believe is worth reporting. The supervised are, according to the qualified nurses, as part of their supervision asked about specific aspects of the patients as they work. They are expected to report any problems or anything unusual to the supervisors.

The Admission Procedure (from the Hospital Procedure Manual)

Admission to hospital

The patient and relatives are welcomed by nursing staff or ward clerk. The patient may be seated or prepared for bed, depending on medical condition.

Relatives or friends are asked to wait until it is ascertained whether the nurse in charge or doctor wishes to see them. Details about visiting are given to relatives and any information required is obtained from them depending on condition of patient.

Documentation and communication

1. Collect and document necessary information required, making sure that it is written legibly and accurately.
2. Make out charts, e.g. temperature charts.
3. Record temperature, pulse, respiration. Record weight and height if required. Specimen of urine is obtained and tested as soon as possible.
4. Identity band with patient's particulars (name, d.o.b., unit no., ward no., hospital) is placed on patient's wrist.
5. Consent for operation is required if patient is for surgery or other therapeutic procedure. This is responsibility of doctor.
6. Patient is asked to undress, and outdoor clothes are given to relatives or stored in appropriate cupboard.
7. Clothes and valuables are documented in the appropriate way.
8. Relatives may see patient before leaving, also nurse in charge or doctor if requested or necessary.
9. Orientate patient to ward and introduce to fellow patients.
10. Care plan and patient profile are compiled.
11. Bath patient if required and if patient appears in a neglected condition hair must be inspected and brushed if necessary.
12. Any medication brought into hospital should be given to nurse in charge.
13. Reassurance for both patient and relatives is very important.

Appendix 7
Nursing Record Charts

NURSING RECORD

WARD   ADMITTING NURSE

Surname	First Names	Next of Kin	Relationship
Address		Address	
			Tel. No.
Tel. No.		Immediate Contact	
Date of Birth	Age Sex	Address	
Marital Status M S W D Sep.	Rel.		Tel. No.
Date of Admission	Time	Day/Night Call	
Source W/L A/E OPD TR GP REF		GP	
Reason for Admission		Address	
Medical Diagnosis			

RELEVANT MEDICAL HISTORY

CURRENT MEDICATIONS

PERSONAL BELONGINGS

	Clothing
	Money
	Valuables

PHYSICAL ASSESSMENT

Gen. Condition	Skin Condition
Ability to Communicate	Allergies
Mobility	Cardio/Resp. Function
HT WT	
Diet	BP T P R
Bladder	Sight/Hearing
Bowel	
Hygiene	Sleep

SOCIAL AND PSYCHOLOGICAL ASSESSMENT

	Occupation
	Social Activities
	Emotional Status
Family Support	
Health Services	HV Dist. Nurse
Physio.	OT Other
Social & Vol. Services	Home Help Soc. Worker
Meals on Wheels	Other

Discharge Date	Home	Convalescence	Transferred	Died
Arrangements	Amb.	OP Appt.	Dist. Nurse	Soc. Worker	Other
Clothing		Valuables		Money

INVESTIGATIONS, OPERATIONS, SPECIAL PROCEDURES

Date Ordered	Procedure	Date Completed	Nurse Signature	Date	Miscellaneous Information

PROGRESS NOTES

Date	Prob. No.	Nursing Action Taken	Progress/Evaluation	Signature

SURNAME   FIRST NAMES   CONSULTANT

NURSING CARE PLAN

Page No.::

Date	Existing/Potential Problems	Short/Long Term Aims	Planned Nursing Action	Evaluate Date/Time	Date Discontinued	Nurse Init.

Appendix 8

Examples of Nursing Records

NAME: *Mr Donald*

NURSING CARE PLAN

Page No.

Date		Existing/Potential Problems	Short/Long Term Aims	Planned Nursing Action	Evaluate Date/Time	Date Discontinued	Nurse Init.
4/4/	①	Obesity	To reduce	i. Commence on reducing diet			
				to be seen by dietician			
		Skin	To maintain	ii. Monitor for pressure sores			
				iii. Clean bd – monitor existing			
				abrasions			
	②	Diabetes	To maintain blood	Monitor blood levels			
			sugar levels	BM stix bd			
	③	Immobility	To prevent	i. Mobilise as able			
			complications of	ii. Use of all aids			
	④	Constipation	To alleviate/prevent	i. Administer suppositories/enemas			
				as prescribed			
	⑤	Hygiene	To maintain	i. Thorough bed bath			
				ii. Basin at bedside as able			
				iii. Big bath as able			
6/4/	⑥	Infected ® arm	To heal	Irrigate with hydrogen peroxide			
				Clean with normal saline			
				Apply Scherisorb and Lycafoam held			
				on with Hypafix			

PROGRESS NOTES

Date	Prob. No.	Nursing Action Taken	Progress/Evaluation	Signature
4/4/			Mr Donald was admitted at 14.30 to ward 2 via A&E. He collapsed this am at his home and lay for 4 hours. His hygiene	
			is poor and he has many abrasions and bruising on ®side where he lay. He smokes 60/day, lives on his own, though	
			has home help. Does not drink. He is a non-insulin dependent diabetic and takes metformin IG tid	
5/4/	(night)	20 turns from back to Ⓛ side	Washed in bed, settled since admission	Staff Nurse
		Incontinent xl of urine	® side painful from falls at home, unable to find bottle	
			in time.	Staff Nurse
	③	Up to sit for afternoon	Required two nurses to transfer.	
			Please encourage patient to help himself.	
	⑤	Washed in bed	All care given	
		BM stix at 6 pm	17 mmol	
		Oral hypoglycaemic given		
		Lactulose prescribed	Complaining of constipation	
		6 pm observations	p120 & T37.3	Staff Nurse
6/4/	(night)	Turned regularly from back to Ⓛ side	Incontinent xl of urine, appears disoriented at times.	
			T37.2 p120 BM 17 at 06.00	Staff Nurse
		Bedbathed fully	Not attempting to help much,	
			has limited use of ® side but	
		Possibly for further investigations	when transferring with two nurses	
			tends to lean to Ⓛ side	Staff Nurse
		Slightly pyrexial	10 am – 37^{-3}, temp 37^4 @ 14.00	Sister

SURNAME *Donald*   FIRST NAMES   CONSULTANT

References

Barker, W.H., Williams, T.F., Zimmer, J.G., Van Buren, C., Vincent, S.J. & Pickrel, S.G. (1985) Geriatric consultation teams in acute hospitals: impact on back-up of elderly patients. *Journal of the American Geriatrics Society*, 33 422–8.

Baruch, G. (1981) Moral tales: parents stories of encounters with the health profession. *Sociology of Health and Illness* 3 (3) 275–96.

Bauman, Z. (1990) Effacing the face. On the social management of moral proximity. *Theory, Culture and Society* 7 (1) 5–38.

Bauman, Z. (1991) The social manipulation of morality: moralizing actors, adiaphorising action. *Theory, Culture and Society* 8 (1) 137–51.

Becker, G. & Kaufman, S.R. (1995) Managing an uncertain illness trajectory in old age: patients' and physicians' views of stroke. *Medical Anthropology Quarterly* 9 (2) 165–87.

Benner, P. (1984) *From Novice to Expert. Excellence and Power in Clinical Nursing Practice*. Addison-Wesley, California.

Benner, P. (1996) The primacy of caring and the role of experience: narrative, and community in clinical and ethical expertise. In *Expertise in Nursing Practice: Caring, Clinical Judgement, and Ethics* (P. Benner, C.A. Tanner & C.A. Chesla, eds), pp. 232–57. Springer Publishing Company, New York.

Benner, P. & Tanner, C. (1987) How expert nurses use intuition. *American Journal of Nursing* 87 23–31.

Benner, P. & Wrubel, J. (1989) *The Primacy of Caring. Stress and Coping in Health and Illness*. Addison-Wesley, California.

Benner, P., Tanner, C. & Chesla, C. (1992) From beginner to expert: gaining a differentiated clinical world in critical care nursing. *Advances in Nursing Science* 14 (3) 13–28.

Berg, M. (1992) The construction of medical disposals. Medical sociology and medical problem-solving in clinical practice. *Sociology of Health and Illness* 14 (2) 151–80.

Berger, P. & Luckmann, T. (1966) *The Social Construction of Reality. A Treatise in the Sociology of Knowledge*. Penguin Books, Harmondsworth.

Bittner, E. (1973). The concept of organisation. In *People and Organisations* (G. Salaman & K. Thompson, eds). Longman/Open University Press, London.

Bloor, M. & McIntosh, J. (1990) Surveillance and concealment: a comparison of techniques of client resistance in therapeutic communities and health visiting. In

Readings in Medical Sociology (S. Cunningham-Burley & N.P. McKeganey, eds). Tavistock/Routledge, London.

Bouchier, I. & Williamson, J. (1982) The elderly patient in the acute hospital sector. *Health Bulletin* **40** (4) 179–82.

Broadbent, J., Laughlin, R. & Read, S. (1991) Recent financial and administrative changes in the NHS: a critical theory analysis. *Critical Perspectives on Accounting* **2** (1) 1–30.

Brocklehurst, J.C. (1978) The evolution of geriatric medicine. *Journal of the American Geriatrics Society* **26** 433–9.

Brocklehurst, J.C. (1982) Health visiting and the elderly: a geriatrician's view. *Health Visitor* **55** 356–7.

Bruni, N. (1995) Reshaping ethnography: contemporary post-positivist possibilities. *Nursing Inquiry* **2** 44–52.

Buckholdt, D.R. & Gubrium, J.F. (1979) Doing staffings. *Human Organisation* **38** (3) 255–64.

Burley, L.E., Currie, C.T., Smith, R.G. & Williamson, J. (1979) Contributions of geriatric medicine within acute medical wards. *British Medical Journal* **2** 90–92.

Coid, J. & Crome, P. (1986) Bed blocking in Bromley. *British Medical Journal* **292** 1253–6.

Crow, R., Chase, J. & Lamond, D. (1995) The cognitive component of nursing assessment: an analysis. *Journal of Advanced Nursing* **22** 206–12.

Currie, C.T., Smith, R.G. & Williamson, J. (1979) Medical and nursing needs of elderly patients admitted to acute medical beds. *Age and Ageing* **8** 149–51.

Davies, C. (1995) *Gender and the Professional Predicament of Nursing*. Open University Press, Buckingham.

Deetz, S. (1992) Disciplinary power in the modern corporation. In *Critical Management Studies* (M. Alvesson & H. Willmott, eds). Sage, London.

Dingwall, R., Rafferty, A.M. & Webster, C. (1988) *An Introduction to the Social History of Nursing*. Routledge, London.

Donaldson, L.J. (1983) Care of the elderly in hospitals and homes: foci of discontent. *Journal of Rehabilitation and Social Health* **5** 181–5.

Douglas, M. (1966) *Purity and Danger. An Analysis of the Concepts of Pollution and Taboo*. Ark Paperbacks, New York.

Fairclough, N. (1992) Discourse and text: linguistic and intertextual analysis within discourse analysis. *Discourse and Society* **3** (2) 193–217.

Faulkner, A. (1985) The organizational context of interpersonal skills in nursing. In *Interpersonal Skills In Nursing. Research and Applications* (C.M. Kagan, ed.). Croom Helm, Kent.

Faulkner, A. & Maguire, P. (1984) Teaching nursing assessment. In *Communication* (A. Faulkner, ed.). Churchill Livingstone, Edinburgh.

Foucault, M. (1976) *The Birth of the Clinic*. Tavistock Publications, London.

Foucault, M. (1979) My body, this paper, this fire. *Oxford Literary Review* **4** (1) 9–28.

Foucault, M. (1980) The masked philosopher. In *Michel Foucault: Politics, Philosophy and Culture. Interviews and Other Writings 1977–1984* (L.D. Kritzman, ed.). Routledge, New York.

Foucault, M. (1991) Politics and the study of discourse. In *The Foucault Effect: Studies in Governmentality* (Burchell, Gordon & Milles, eds). Harvester Wheatsheaf, London.

Garfinkel, H. (1967) *Studies in Ethnomethodology*. Prentice-Hall, Englewood Cliffs.

Garfinkel, H. & Sacks, H. (1969) On formal structures of practical actions. In *Ethnomethodological Studies of Work* (H. Garfinkel, ed.). Routledge and Kegan Paul, London.

Geertz, C. (1995) *After the Fact*. Harvard University Press, Boston.

Giddens, A. (1984) *The Constitution of Society. Outline of Structuration Theory*. Polity Press, Cambridge.

Giddens, A. (1991) *Modernity and Self-Identity*. Polity Press, Cambridge.

Gilbert, N. & Mulkay, M. (1983) In search of the action. In *Accounts and Action. Surrey Conference on Social Theory and Method* (G.N. Gilbert & P. Abell, eds). Gower, Aldershot.

Gillick, M.R., Sewell, N.A. & Gillick, L.S. (1982) Adverse consequences of hospitalization in the elderly. *Social Science and Medicine* 16 1033–8.

Goffman, E. (1958) *The Presentation of Self in Everyday Life*. University of Edinburgh, Social Sciences Research Centre, Monograph No. 2.

Goffman, E. (1978) On the characteristics of total institutions. In *Modern Sociology* (P. Worsley, ed.). Penguin Books Ltd, Harmondsworth.

Green, J. & Armstrong, D. (1993) Controlling the bedstate: negotiating hospital organisation. *Sociology of Health and Illness* 15(3) 337–352.

Gregor, F. (1997) From women to women: nurses, informal caregivers and the gender dimension of health care reform. *Health and Social Care in the Community* 5 (1) 30–36.

Hamdy, R.C. (1984) *Geriatric Medicine. A Problem-Orientated Approach*. Baillière Tindall, London.

Henderson, V. (1981) The nursing process: is the title right? *Journal of Advanced Nursing* 7 103–9.

Hetherington, K. & Munro, R. (eds) (1997) *Ideas of Difference: Social Spaces and the Labour of Division*. Sociological Review Monograph. Blackwell Publishers, Oxford.

Hiraki, A. (1992) Tradition, rationality and power in introductory nursing textbooks: a critical hermeneutics study. *Advances in Nursing Science* 14 (3) 1–12.

Hulter Asberg, K.H. (1986) *Elderly patients in acute medical wards and home care. Functional assessment, prediction of outcome, and a trial of early activation*. PhD Thesis, University of Uppsala, Sweden.

Hurst, K. & Dean, A. (1987) An Investigation into Nurses' Perceptions of Problem-Solving in Clinical Practice. Proceedings of Nursing Research Congress. *Clinical Excellence in Nursing, International Networking*.

Hurst, K., Dean, A. & Trickey, S. (1991) The recognition and non-recognition of problem-solving stages in nursing practice. *Journal of Advanced Nursing* 16 1444–55.

Jolley, D.J. (1987) *The Aetiology of Confusion*. Presentation given at the British

Journal of Hospital Medicine Conference: The Care of the Elderly Patient in the Acute Medical Unit, Edinburgh.

King's Fund (1982) *The Respective Roles of the General Acute and Geriatric Sectors in the Care of the Elderly Hospitalised Patient.* Report of a Study Day held on 4th June 1982. KFC 82/213.

Latimer, J. (1994) *Writing Patients, Writing Nursing: The Social Construction of Nursing Assessment of Elderly Patients in an Acute Medical Unit.* PhD Thesis, University of Edinburgh.

Latimer, J. (1995) The nursing process re-examined: diffusion or translation? *Journal of Advanced Nursing* **22** 213–20.

Latimer, J. (1997) Giving patients a future: the constituting of classes in an acute medical unit. *Sociology of Health and Illness* **19** (2) 160–85.

Latimer, J. (1999) The dark at the bottom of the stair: participation and performance of older people in hospital. *Medical Anthropology Quarterly* **13** (2) 186–213.

Latour, B. (1991) Technology is society made durable. In *A Sociology of Monsters* (J. Law, ed.). Sociological Review Monograph 38. Blackwell, Oxford.

Lawler, J. (1991) *Behind the Screens. Nursing, Somology, and the Problem of the Body.* Churchill Livingstone, Edinburgh.

Lentz, E. (1954) *A Comparison of Medical and Surgical Floors.* Mimeograph: New York State School of Industrial and Labour Relations, Cornell University.

Lupton, D. (1996) *Medicine as Culture. Illness, Disease and the Body in Western Societies.* Sage, London.

Lyth, I.M. (1960) Social systems as a defense against anxiety. An empirical study of the nursing service of a general hospital. In *The Social Engagement of Social Science. Volume 1. The Socio-psychological Perspective* (E. Trist & H. Murray, eds). Free Association Books, London.

McArdle, C., Wylie, J.C. & Alexander, W.D. (1975) Geriatric patients in an acute medical ward. *British Medical Journal* **4** 568–9.

Mackay, L. (1989) *Nursing a Problem.* Open University Press, Milton Keynes.

MacLennan, W.J. (1987) *Ageing.* Presentation at the British Journal of Hospital Medicine Conference. The Care of the Elderly Patient in the Acute Medical Unit. Edinburgh.

Marcus, G. & Fischer, M. (1986) *Anthropology as Cultural Critique: An Experimental Moment in the Human Sciences.* Chicago University Press, Chicago.

May, C. (1991) *Getting to know them: an exploratory study of nurses' relationships and work with terminally ill patients in acute medical and surgical wards.* PhD Thesis, University of Edinburgh.

May, C. (1992) Individual care? Power and subjectivity in therapeutic relationships. *Sociology* **26** (4) 589–602.

Melia, K. (1981) *Student nurses' accounts of their work and training: a qualitative analysis.* PhD Thesis, University of Edinburgh.

Miller, A. (1984) Nurse/patient dependency – a review of different approaches with particular reference to studies of the dependency of elderly patients. *Journal of Advanced Nursing* **9** 479–86.

Morrison, E.G. (1989) Nursing assessment: what do nurses want to know? *Western Journal of Nursing Research* 11 (4) 469–76.

Mueller, M. (1995) *Organising participation: an ethnography of 'community' in hospital*. PhD Thesis, University of Edinburgh.

Munro, R. (1996) Alignments and identity-work: the study of accounts and accountability. In *Accountability: Power, Ethos and the Technologies of Managing* (R. Munro and J. Mouritsen, eds). Thomson International Press, London.

Osterwalder, H. (1978) *T.S. Eliot: Between Metaphor and Metonomy. A Study of His Essays and Plays in Terms of Roman Jakobson's Typology*. Francke Verlag, Berne.

Pearson, A. & Vaughn, B. (1986) *Nursing Models for Practice*. Heinemann Nursing, London.

Peterson, W.A. (1985) Preface. In *Social Bonds In Later Life. Ageing and Interdependence* (W.A. Peterson & J. Quadagno, eds). Sage, Beverly Hills.

Price, R. (1987) First impressions: paradigms for patient assessment. *Journal of Advanced Nursing* 13 699–705.

Purkis, M.E. (1993) *Bringing 'practice' to the clinic: an excavation of the effects of health promotion discourse on nursing practice in a community health clinic*. PhD Thesis, University of Edinburgh.

Purkis, M.E. (1996) Nursing in quality space: technologies governing experiences of care. *Nursing Inquiry* 3 101–11.

Rafferty, A.M. (1996) *The Politics of Nursing Knowledge*. Routledge, London.

Roper, N., Logan, W. & Tierney, A. (1980) *The Elements of Nursing*. Churchill Livingstone, Edinburgh.

Roper, N., Logan, W. & Tierney, A. (1981) *Learning to Use the Nursing Process*. Churchill Livingstone, Edinburgh.

Rose, N. & Miller, P. (1992) Political power beyond the state: problematics of government. *British Journal of Sociology* 43 (2) 173–205.

Rubin, S.G. & Davies, G.H. (1975) Bed blocking by elderly patients in general hospital wards. *Age and Ageing* 4 142–7.

Rudge, T. (1996) (Re) writing ethnography: the unsettling questions for nursing raised by post-structural approaches to the field. *Nursing Inquiry* 3 146–52.

Rudge, T. (1997) *Nursing wounds: a discourse analysis of nurse–patient interactions during wound care procedures in a burns unit*. PhD Thesis, La Trobe University, Melbourne.

Salvage, J. (1992) The new nursing: empowering patients or empowering nurses? In *Policy Issues in Nursing* (J. Robinson, A. Gray & R. Elkan, eds). Open University, Milton Keynes.

Seymour, D.G. & Pringle, R. (1982) Elderly patients in general surgical units: do they block beds? *British Medical Journal* 284 1921–3.

Silverman, D. (1987) *Communication and Medical Practice. Social Relations in the Clinic*. Sage, London.

Silverman, D. (1989) The impossible dreams of reformism and romanticism. In *The Politics of Field Research: Sociology Beyond Enlightenment* (D. Silverman & J. Gubrium, eds). Sage, London.

Silverman, D. (1993) *Interpreting Qualitative Data. Methods for Analysing Talk, Text and Interaction.* Sage, London.

Stevens, W. (1947) *Transport to Summer.* AA Kopf, New York.

Strathern, M. (1991) *Partial Connections.* Rowman and Littlefield Publishers, Maryland.

Strathern, M. (1992) Writing societies, writing persons. *History of Human Sciences* **5** (1) 5–16.

Strathern, M. (1993) Society in drag. *Times Higher Educational Supplement*, 2 April p. 19.

Strathern, M. (1995) *The Relation. Issues in Complexity and Scale.* Prickly Pear Press, Cambridge.

Strathern, M. (1997) Gender: comparison or division? In *Ideas of Difference: Social Space and the Labour of Division.* Sociological Review Monograph. Blackwell Publishers, Oxford.

Strong, P. & Robinson, J. (1990) *The NHS Under New Management.* Open University Press, Milton Keynes.

Tanner, C., Padrick, K., Westfall, U. & Putzier, D. (1987) Diagnostic reasoning strategies of nurses and nursing students. *Nursing Research* **36** (6) 358–63.

Thiele, J.E., Holloway, J., Murphy, D., Pendarvis, J. & Stucky, M. (1991) Perceived and actual decision making by novice baccalaureate students. *Western Journal of Nursing Research* **13** (5) 616-26.

Tierney, A.J. (1984) A response to Professor Mitchell's 'simple guide to the nursing process'. *British Medical Journal* **288** 835–8.

Tilley, S. (1995) *Negotiating Realities: Making Sense of Interaction between Patients Diagnosed as Neurotic and Nurses in Two Psychiatric Admissions Wards.* Ashgate, Avebury.

Turner, V. (1967) *The Forest of Symbols: Aspects of Ndembu Ritual.* Cornell University Press, New York.

Victor, C. & Vetter, N.J. (1984) DNs and the elderly after hospital discharge. *Nursing Times* **80** (15) 61–2.

Walton, I. (1986) *The Nursing Process in Perspective. A Literature Review.* Department of Social Policy and Social Work, University of York.

Ward, M. (1988) Sociolinguistics and the nursing process. *Senior Nurse* **8** (11) 21–3.

Wells, T. (1980) *Problems in Geriatric Nursing Care.* Churchill Livingstone, Edinburgh.

Index